Air Fryer Cookbook

Over 150+ Delicious Recipes Including Vegan
Friendly Options!

Table of Contents

The following book is reproduced below with the goal of providing information that is as accurate and reliable as possible. Regardless, purchasing this book can be seen as consent to the fact that both the publisher and the author of this book are in no way experts on the topics discussed within and that any recommendations or suggestions that are made herein are for entertainment purposes only. Professionals should be consulted as needed prior to undertaking any of the action endorsed herein.

This declaration is deemed fair and valid by both the American Bar Association and the Committee of Publishers Association and is legally binding throughout the United States.

Furthermore, the transmission, duplication or reproduction of any of the following work including specific information will be considered an illegal act irrespective of if it is done electronically or in print. This extends to creating a secondary or tertiary copy of the work or a recorded copy and is only allowed with an expressed written consent from the Publisher. All additional rights reserved.

The information in the following pages is broadly considered to be truthful and accurate account of facts, and as such any inattention, use or misuse of the information in question by the reader will render any resulting actions solely under their

Introduction

Congratulations and thank you for purchasing this book. Air Frying is genuinely one of the easiest and fastest ways to fry your food. The lack of oil ensures you aren't consuming an excess of harmful fat. Did you know though that an air fryer can be used for purposes other than just frying?

The air fryer does so much more than just frying. Its repertoire includes grilling, baking, steaming, and roasting. From eggs to desserts, it is all delicious. This book has special sections dedicated to vegan and vegetarian diet plans and the recipes therein are guaranteed to tickle your taste buds!

There are plenty of books on this subject on the market, thanks again for choosing this one!

Please do leave a review on Amazon if you found this book useful in any way at all!

Chapter 1: Delicious Breakfast & Brunch Choices

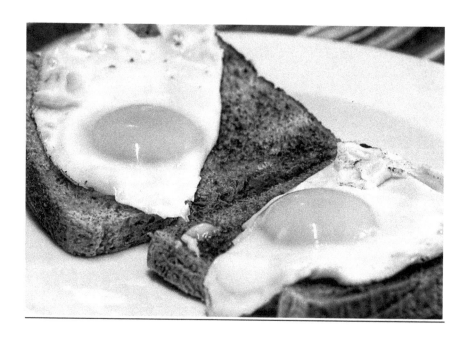

Super Eggs

Avocado Egg Boats

Yields: 2 Servings

Ingredients:

1 avocado

2 large eggs

To Taste:

 -Chives

 -Parsley

 -Pepper

 -Salt

Preparation Steps:

1. Program the Air Fryer to 350°F.
2. Cut the avocado in half, discard the pit to make room for the mixture. Add in the salt and pepper.
3. Add an egg to each half and place in the Air Fryer for six minutes.
4. Serve with some freshly chopped parsley and chives if desired.

Bacon and Eggs

Ingredients:

4 eggs

12 slices of bacon - 1/2-inch thickness

Pepper and salt

1 tbsp. butter

2 sliced croissants

4 tbsp. softened butter

Ingredients for the Barbecue Sauce:

2 tbsp. each:

  -Molasses

  -Brown sugar

¼ c. apple cider vinegar

1 c. ketchup

½ tsp. each:

  -Onion powder

  -Mustard powder

  - Liquid smoke

1 tbsp. Worcestershire sauce

Preparation Steps:

1. Warm up the Air Fryer to 390°F.
2. Make the barbecue sauce by combining the molasses, ketchup, brown sugar, vinegar, onion powder, and mustard powder in a soup pot over medium heat on the stove.

3. Whisk the liquid smoke and Worcestershire sauce into the mixture. Blend thoroughly. Cook until the sauce thickens. Add additional flavoring as desired.
4. Arrange the bacon on the Air Fryer trays and cook for 5 minutes. Remove and brush the bacon with the barbecue sauce, flip, and brush the other side. Return the bacon in the Air Fryer and continue cooking another 5 minutes.
5. Butter the halved croissant and toast it in the fryer.
6. While you are waiting, on the stove top, use a non-stick pan on the med-low setting to melt the butter. Add 4 eggs and cook until the white starts setting. Flip and cook about thirty more seconds.
7. Remove from the pan and enjoy with the bacon and croissant.

Bacon & Egg Cups

Yields: 4 Servings

Ingredients:

4 eggs
½ tsp. of each:
-Paprika

-Dried dill

¼ tsp. salt

6 oz. bacon

1 tbsp. butter

Also Needed: 4 ramekins

Preparation Steps:

1. Warm up the Air Fryer to 360°F.
2. Using a hand mixer, whisk the eggs then add the salt, paprika, and dried dill
3. Coat the ramekins with butter.
4. Slice the bacon and use it to line the inside of the cups. Pour the egg mixture into the center of each cup and cook for 15 minutes.
5. Gently remove the cups and serve.

Bread Bowl Baked Eggs

Yields: 4 Egg Bowls

Ingredients:

4 dinner rolls – crusty

4 large eggs

4 tbsp. of each:

-Heavy cream

-Grated parmesan cheese

-Mixed herbs – for ex. Chopped tarragon, chives, parsley, etc.

Preparation Steps:

1. Preheat the Air Fryer until it reaches 350°F.
2. Cut off the top of each of the rolls, set the top aside. Scoop out some bread to form a hole at the center, large enough for the egg.
3. Place the rolls in the fryer basket. Break an egg into the roll and top with the cream and chosen herbs. Sprinkle with some parmesan.
4. Bake for 20 to 25 minutes until the egg is set, and the bread toasted.
5. Arrange the tops of the bread on the egg and bake a minute or so to finish the browning process.
6. Let the eggs rest for 5 minutes. Serve warm.

Egg Pizza

Yields: 1 Serving

Ingredients:

2 eggs

½ tsp. dried of each:

 -Basil

-Oregano

2 tbsp. shredded mozzarella cheese

4 thin slices of pepperoni

Also Needed: 1 ramekin

Preparation Steps:

1. Whisk the eggs with the oregano and basil.
2. Pour into the ramekin and top off with the pepperoni and cheese.
3. Arrange the ramekin in the Air Fryer. Cook for 3 minutes and enjoy.

Ham & Eggs with Spinach

Yields: 4 Servings

Ingredients:

2 ¼ c. spinach

7 oz. sliced ham

4 large eggs

4 tsp. milk

1 tbsp. olive oil

To Your Liking: Pepper & Salt

Also Needed: 4 Ramekins

Preparation Steps:

1. Program the fryer temperature to 356°F.
2. Spray the ramekins.
3. Warm up the oil in a skillet using the medium heat setting. Sauté the spinach until wilted. Drain.
4. Divide the spinach and the rest of the fixings in each of the ramekins. Sprinkle with the salt and pepper.
5. Bake until set or about 20 minutes.
6. Serve and enjoy.

Scrambled Eggs

Yields: 1 Serving

Ingredients:

2 eggs

Pepper and salt to taste

Preparation Steps:

1. Warm up the Air Fryer to 284ºF (5 min.).
2. Put the butter in the fryer to melt and spread it out evenly.
3. Break the eggs into the fryer and add other ingredients such as cheese or tomatoes if you desire.
4. Open the fryer every few minutes to whisk the eggs for the desired, fluffy consistency.
5. Serve with toast on the side or enjoy a scrambled egg sandwich.

Tasty Spinach Frittata

Yields: 1-2 Servings

Ingredients:

1 small minced red onion

1/3 pkg. of spinach

A sprinkle of Mozzarella cheese

3 eggs

Preparation Steps:

1. Program the temperature of the Air Fryer to 356°F for at least 3 minutes.
2. Pour the oil into the Air Fryer baking pan to warm up for 1 minute.
3. Toss in the onions. Cook for 2 to 3 minutes.
4. Add in spinach and cook for 3 to 5 minutes.
5. Whisk in the eggs and add the seasonings and cheese to the pan.
6. Air fry for 8 minutes. Give it a shake of pepper and salt.

Sweet Treats

Apple Dumplings

Yields: 2 Servings

Ingredients:

2 small apples
2 tbsp. of each:
  -Melted butter
  -Raisins
1 tbsp. brown sugar
2 sheets puff pastry

Tip: Be sure to use tiny apples for this yummy treat.

Preparation Steps:

1. Peel and core the apples.
2. Program the Air Fryer to 356°F.
3. In a bowl, mix the sugar and raisins.
4. Arrange each apple on one of the pastry sheets and fill each cored apple with the raisins-sugar mixture. Fold the pastry over until the apple and raisins are adequately covered.
5. Thoroughly brush with the melted butter.
6. Place them on a piece of foil so they do not fall through the fryer.
7. Air fry for 25 minutes and serve.

Apple Steel-Cut Oats

Yields: 6 Servings

Ingredients:

2 apples

1 c. steel-cut oats

1 tbsp. ground flaxseed

1 1/2 c. of each:

 -Coconut milk

 -Water

2 tsp. of each:

  -Vanilla extract

  -Stevia

1/2 tsp. cinnamon

1/4 tsp. ground of each:

 -Cardamom

 -Ginger powder

 -Allspice

 -Nutmeg

Preparation Steps:

1. Core, peel, and chop the apples.
2. Warm up the Air Fryer until it reaches 360°F.
3. Lightly coat the fryer with some cooking spray.
4. Add the apples with the rest of the ingredients in the fryer bucket.
5. Set the timer for 15 minutes. Serve when ready.

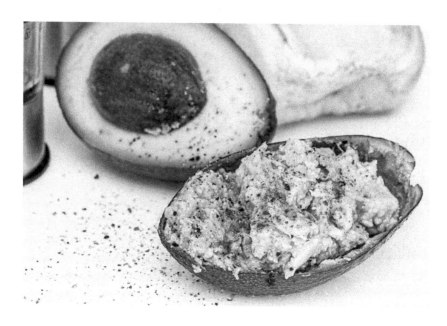

Avocado Muffins

Yields: 7 Servings

Ingredients:

1 c. almond flour

1 tsp. apple cider vinegar

½ tsp. baking soda

2 tsp. of stevia powder

1 oz. melted dark chocolate

1 egg

4 tbsp. butter

½ c. avocado

Preparation Steps

1. Preheat the Air Fryer to 355°F.
2. Whisk the vinegar with the baking soda and almond flour. Add the stevia powder and melted chocolate. Then add in the whisked egg and butter.
3. Peel, cube, and mash the avocado then add to the mixture. Blend with a hand mixer to make the mixture smooth.
4. Pour into the muffin tin until half full. Cook for 9 minutes.
5. Lower the heat to 340°F and cook 3 more minutes.
6. Cool before serving.

Banana Fritters

Yields: 6-8 Servings

Ingredients:

8 ripe- peeled bananas

3 tbsp. corn flour

1 egg white

3 tbsp. vegetable oil

¾ c. breadcrumbs

Preparation Steps:

1. Set the temperature of the Air Fryer to 356°F.
2. In a skillet using the low heat setting, pour the oil and toss in the breadcrumbs, cooking until golden brown.
3. Use the corn flour to coat the bananas then dip them into the egg white and cover with the breadcrumbs.
4. Place the bananas in a single layer of the basket and cook for 8 minutes.
5. Remove and drain on paper towels.

Banana & Walnut Oats

Yields: 4 Servings

Ingredients:

1 banana

1/4 c. chopped walnuts

1 c. steel-cut oats

2 c. of each:

  -Almond milk

  -Water

2 tbsp. flaxseed meal

2 t cinnamon

1 tsp. vanilla extract

1/2 tsp. ground nutmeg

Preparation Steps:

1. Set the temperature of the Air Fryer to 360°F to preheat.
2. Peel and mash the banana. Chop the walnuts and combine with all the ingredients.
3. Mix well and cook for 15 minutes.
4. Serve and enjoy when ready.

Choco Zucchini Bread

Yields: 12 Servings

Ingredients:

1 tbsp. flax meal

3 tbsp. water

1 c. of each:

 -Zucchini

 -Oat flour

1/2 c. of each:

 -Maple syrup

-Sunflower oil

-Almond milk

-Unsweetened cocoa powder

1/3 c. chocolate chips

1 tsp. of each:

-Apple cider vinegar

-Vanilla extract

-Baking soda

1/4 tsp. salt

Preparation Steps:

1. Make a flax egg by combining 1 tablespoon of flax meal and with 3 tablespoons of water.
2. Cut the zucchini into strips and place in a microwave-safe bowl. Place the zucchini in the microwave on high for 5 minutes.   Remove as much liquid from it as possible.
3. Preheat the Air Fryer to 350°F.
4. Line the baking dish with parchment paper.
5. Combine the 1 tbsp. flax egg, oil, vanilla, zucchini, maple syrup, milk, and vinegar. Add the dry ingredients (salt, cocoa, baking soda, and oat flour).
6. Mix well and fold in the chocolate chips.

7. Pour into the baking dish and cook for 15 minutes. Perform the toothpick test to see if its done. The toothpick should come out clean.

8. Serve and enjoy!

Cranberry Coconut Quinoa

Yields: 4 Servings

Ingredients:

1/4 c. dried cranberries

1/8 c. chopped almonds

1/8 c. coconut flakes

3 tsp. stevia

1 c. quinoa

3 c. coconut water

1 tsp. vanilla extract

Preparation Steps:

1. Warm up the Air Fryer to 365°F.
2. Chop the almonds and combine with the rest of the ingredients.
3. Pour into the fryer basket.

4. Cook for 13 minutes.

5. Enjoy!

French Toast Sticks

Yields: 2 Servings

Ingredients:

4 slices of bread of choice

2 eggs

2 tbsp. soft margarine or butter

A pinch of each:

   -Salt

   -Cinnamon

   -Ground cloves

   -Nutmeg

For topping: Maple syrup or Whipped cream

Preparation Steps:

1. Set the temperature of the Air Fryer to 356°F.

2. Whisk the eggs and add a shake of nutmeg, cloves, and cinnamon.

3. Spread butter on both sides of the bread and cut them into strips. Dredge each of the pieces in the egg mixture then arrange and cook in the fryer.
4. Pause the fryer after 2 minutes, remove the pan, and spray the bread with cooking spray.
5. Flip and spray the other side, then return them to the fryer to cook for an additional 4 minutes. Ensure they do not burn. It's ready when it is golden brown.
6. Garnish with some maple syrup or whipped cream. Drizzle some confectioner's sugar for a sweeter experience. Serve immediately.

Mixed Berry Muffins

Yields: 8 Muffins

Ingredients:

1 c. mixed berries of your choice

2 tsp. baking powder

1 1/3 c. and 1 tbsp. flour

1/4 c. white sugar

2 tbsp. brown sugar

2/3 c. whole milk

1/3 c. safflower oil

2 eggs

Also Needed: 8 Foil muffin cups

Preparation Steps:

1. Set the temperature of the Air Fryer to 320°F.
2. Combine the baking powder, brown sugar, white sugar, and 1 1/3 cups of the flour.
3. In another bowl, combine the oil, eggs, and milk. Whisk well.
4. Combine the two mixtures together until it slightly mixed.
5. Coat the berries with the 1 tbsp. flour.
6. Add the berries into the batter gently.
7. Arrange 4 cups in the Air Fryer (3/4 full).
8. Bake until the muffins are done which is about 12-17 minutes.
9. Make the second batch the same way.
10. Cool for 10 minutes before serving.

Pear Oatmeal

Yields: 3 Servings

Ingredients:

1 chopped pear

1/2 c. steel-cut oats

2 c. coconut milk

1 tbsp. stevia

1/2 tsp. of each:

  -Vanilla extract

  -Maple extract

Preparation Steps:

1. Set the Air Fryer to 360°F.
2. Combine all the ingredients. Mix well.
3. Add to the fryer and cook for 15 minutes.
4. Serve in three portions and enjoy.

More Yummy Dishes

Bacon & Cheese Muffins

Yields: 6 Servings

Ingredients:

1 large egg

4 thick-cut slices of bacon

1 med. diced onion

2 tbsp. olive oil

2 tsp. baking powder

1 tsp. parsley

1 c. of each:

 -Milk

 -Shredded cheddar cheese

1 ½ c. almond flour

Pepper and salt to taste

Also Needed: 6 muffin tins to fit in the basket

Preparation Steps:

1. Set the temperature on the Air Fryer to 356°F.
2. Prepare the bacon slices in a frying pan with a small amount of oil. Add the onion when the bacon about 3/4 ready. Sauté and set aside once the onion is translucent. Drain on towels. When cooled, break the bacon into bits.
3. In a bowl, mix the rest of the ingredients well. Add the sautéed onions and bacon.
4. Add the batter into 6 muffin holders. Cook in the fryer basket for 20 minutes. Then lower the heat to 320°F and cook for an additional 10 minutes.
5. Serve and enjoy right out of the fryer.

Bacon-Wrapped Tater Tots

Yields: 4 Servings

Ingredients:

3 tbsp. sour cream

1 lb. sliced bacon

1 large bag crispy tater tots

4 scallions

½ c. shredded cheddar cheese

Preparation Steps:

1. Set the temperature of the Air Fryer to 400°F.
2. Wrap each of the tots with bacon and arrange them in the fryer basket. Don't overcrowd, keep them in a single layer.
3. Set the Air Fryer for 8 minutes.
4. When the timer beeps, arrange them on a serving platter or divide into four portions.
5. Serve with the scallions and cheese garnish. Add a dash of sour cream and enjoy.

Cheddar & Bacon Mini Quiche

Yields: 4 Servings

Ingredients:

1/2 c. grated cheddar cheese

3 tbsp. Greek yogurt

3 oz. chopped bacon

4 eggs

1/4 tsp. of each:

  -Garlic powder

  -Salt

  -Onion powder

Pinch of black pepper

Flour for sprinkling

1 Short-crust pastry (see below)

Ingredients for the Pastry Dough:

1 c. All-purpose flour

1 Stick or 1/4 lb. unsalted butter

1/2 tsp. kosher salt

3 tbsp. ice water

Also Needed: 8 Ramekins

Preparation Steps:

Prepare the Dough:

1. Combine the salt and flour in a mixer or food processor.
2. Dice the butter into 1/8-inch pieces then add. Pulse until coarse.
3. Pour in the cold water to form a soft dough.
4. Shape into a disk and refrigerate in plastic wrap overnight or at least two hours in the fridge.
5. Let it come to room temperature before rolling it out.

Make the Quiche:

1. Warm up the fryer until it reaches 330°F.
2. Grease the ramekins and dust with the flour. Tap out the excess flour.
3. Portion the pasty into 8 pieces and arrange in each of the ramekins.
4. Combine the ingredients in a bowl. Mix well. Pour into the prepared crust and place in the fryer.
5. Bake for 20 minutes and serve.

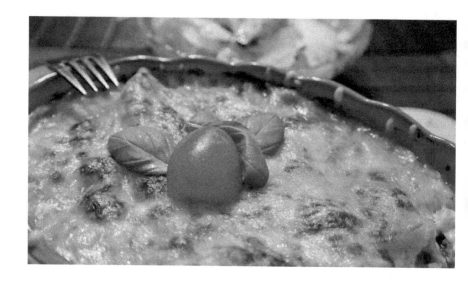

Cheese & Onion Nuggets

Yields: 4 Servings

Ingredients:

1 egg

7 oz. grated Edam cheese

2 diced spring onions

Salt and pepper

1 tbsp. of each:

-Dried thyme

-Coconut oil

Preparation Steps:

1. Preheat the frying unit to 350°F.
2. Combine all the ingredients except for the cheese and egg.
3. Make 8 balls out of the mixture and stuff in the cheese at the center.
4. Place in the fridge for 1 hour.
5. Whisk the egg and use a pastry brush to coat each nugget.
6. Place in the Air Fryer for 12 minutes. Serve.

Rice Paper Bacon

Yields: 4 Servings

Ingredients:

4 pieces of rice paper

3 tbsp. tamari or soy sauce

2 tbsp. of each:

  -Liquid smoke

  -Cashew butter

  -Water

Preparation Steps:

1. Cut the rice paper into 1-inch strips.

2. Warm the Air Fryer to 350°F.

3. Combine the cashew butter, liquid smoke, soy sauce, and water.

4. Soak the rice paper in the mixture for 5 minutes and place in the fryer. Don't let them overlap.

5. Air fry for 15 minutes or until they're the way you like them.

6. Serve with your favorite steamed veggies.

Sausage Wraps

Yields: 8 Wraps

Ingredients:

1 can (8-count) crescent roll dough

2 slices American cheese

8 Heat & Serve Sausages

8 wooden skewers

For Dipping: Ketchup, or barbecue sauce, syrup

Preparation Steps:

1. Set the Air Fryer temperature setting to 380°F.

2. Do the Prep: Slice the cheese into four triangles. Open the sausages and separate the rolls.

3. Add the cheese strips starting from the base of the triangle to the tip. Add the sausage. Pull up each of the ends of the roll over the sausage and cheese. Be sure to pinch all sides together.
4. Cook for 3 to 4 minutes, depending on how crispy you like the bread. Cook in 2 batches
5. Remove from the fryer and add a skewer. Top it off to your liking.

Shrimp Toast

Yields: 4 Servings

Ingredients:

4-5 white bread slices

3/4 lb. raw shrimp

1 egg white

2 tbsp. of each:

  -Cornstarch

  -Olive oil

3 minced garlic cloves

Pepper and salt to taste

Preparation Steps:

1. Peel and devein the shrimp. Mince the cloves of garlic and shrimp.

2. Warm the Air Fryer to 370°F.

3. Whisk the egg white, garlic, cornstarch, pepper, salt, then add in the chopped shrimp.

4. Spread over the slices of bread and spritz with some olive oil.

5. Add the bread slices to the Air Fryer Basket and cook for 10 minutes or until it's lightly browned.

Chapter 2: Tasty Lunches!

Poultry

Buffalo Chicken Wings

Yields: 2-3 Servings

Ingredients:

5 chicken wings

½ tsp. garlic powder - optional

2 tsp. cayenne pepper

1 tbsp. melted butter

2 tbsp. red hot sauce

Black pepper and salt to taste

Preparation Steps:

1. Warm up the Air Fryer at 356°F for about 5 minutes until heated.
2. Cut the wings into three sections (the end tip, middle joint, and drumette). Pat each one thoroughly dry using a paper towel.
3. Combine salt, garlic powder, cayenne pepper and a dash of pepper, in a plate. Lightly coat the wings with the powder.
4. Arrange the wings on the wire rack and bake for 15 minutes. Flip once halfway through the cycle.
5. Combine the hot sauce and melted butter in a dish to garnish the baked chicken when it is time to be served.

    Tip: You can add more cayenne pepper if you want it hotter.

Chicken Curry

Yields: 4 Servings

Ingredients:

1 onion

2 tsp. minced garlic

1 lb. chicken breast – no skin or bones

1 tsp. olive oil

1 tbsp. of each:

-Lemongrass

-Apple cider vinegar

½ c. each:

-Coconut milk

-Chicken stock

2 tbsp. curry paste

Preparation Steps:

1. Warm up the Air Fryer to 365°F.
2. Chop the chicken into cubes.
3. Peel and dice the onion and put into the Air Fryer basket. Cook 5 minutes.
4. Remove the onion, then add the rest of the ingredients into the basket. Mix well and for cook another 10 minutes.
5. Serve and enjoy.

Chicken Escalope

Yields: 4 Servings

Ingredients:

4 skinless breasts of chicken

2 eggs

6 sage leaves

1/2 c. all-purpose flour

1/4 c. of each:

 -Parmesan cheese

 -Panko breadcrumbs

For Spritzing: Oil

Preparation Steps:

1. Preheat the Air Fryer to 390°F.
2. Using a meat mallet, flatten the chicken and cut into thin slices.
3. Combine the flour with the parmesan, salt, pepper, and sage.
4. Whisk the eggs.
5. Dip the chicken into the flour mixture then the eggs and lastly cover with the breadcrumbs.
6. Lightly spritz the pan with oil.
7. Cook the chicken for 20 minutes and enjoy with your favorite side dish.

Chicken Hash

Yields: 3 Servings

Ingredients:

7 oz. chicken fillet

6 oz. chopped cauliflower

½ yellow diced onion

1 chopped green pepper

1 tbsp. of each:

  -Water

  -Cream

1 tsp. black pepper

3 tbsp. butter

Preparation Steps:

1. Heat up the Air Fryer to 380°F.
2. Chop the cauliflower and put in a blender to make cauliflower rice.
3. Dice the onion and the green pepper and chop the chicken into chunks. Add a little pepper and salt.
4. Combine the ingredients in the fryer basket and cook until done (about 6-7 min.). Check often.
5. Serve and enjoy.

Chicken Pot Pie

Yields: 4 Servings

Ingredients:

6 chicken tenders

2 potatoes

1 ½ c. condensed cream of celery soup

¾ c. heavy cream

1 whole bay leaf

1 thyme sprig

5 refrigerated buttermilk biscuits

1 tbsp. milk

1 egg yolk

Preparation Steps:

1. Program the temperature setting on the Air Fryer to 320°F.
2. Remove the skin from the potatoes and dice.
3. Combine the ingredients in a pan except for the milk, egg yolk, and biscuits. Mix and bring to a boil at medium heat setting.
4. Put the mixture into the baking tin and use an aluminum foil to cover the top. Place the baking tin into the fryer basket. Cook for 15 minutes.
5. Meanwhile, make an egg wash by mixing the milk and egg yolk.
6. Place the biscuits on a baking pan and brush them with the egg wash mixture.

7. Set the fryer to 300°F for an additional 10 minutes and cook until it's golden brown.

Chicken Quesadillas

Yields: 4 Servings

Ingredients:

2 tbsp. olive oil - divided

2 soft taco shells

1 lb. boneless chicken breasts

1 med. onion

1 large green pepper

1/2 c. of each:

  -Salsa sauce

  -Shredded cheddar cheese

To Taste: Pepper and Salt

Preparation Steps:

1. Program the Air Fryer to 370°F. Spritz with 1 tbsp. of the oil.
2. Arrange one taco shell in the fryer. On top of it, add a layer of salsa then strips of chicken. Add the peppers and onion with a sprinkle of salt and pepper...

3. Sprinkle with cheese and cover with another shell.
4. Sprinkle with the rest of the oil and secure with the rack to hold the taco in place as it cooks.
5. Set the timer for 4-6 minutes. Slice when done.
6. Serve either hot or cold. Enjoy.

Chicken Tenders - Country-Style

Yields: 4 Servings

Ingredients:

3/4 lb. chicken tenders

½ tsp. salt

2 tbsp. olive oil

2 beaten eggs

½ c. of each:

 -All-purpose flour

 -Seasoned breadcrumbs

1 tsp. black pepper

Preparation Steps:

1. Program the Air Fryer heat setting to 330°F.
2. Prepare three separate dishes for the flour, eggs, and breadcrumbs.

3. Combine the salt, pepper, and breadcrumbs. Pour in the oil with the breadcrumbs. Mix well.

4. Put the chicken tenders into the flour then the eggs. Lastly, coat evenly with the breadcrumbs. Shake the excess coating off before placing in the Air Fryer basket.

5. Cook for 10 minutes at 330°F then increase to 390°F for 5 minutes or until they are golden brown.

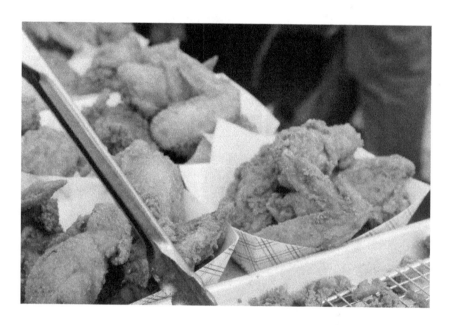

Chinese Chicken Wings

Yields: 2 Servings

Ingredients:

4 chicken wings

Salt and pepper to taste

1 tbsp. each:

-Chinese spice

-Mixed spice

-Soy sauce

Preparation Steps:

1. Warm up the fryer to 356ºF.
2. Add the seasonings into a large mixing container—stir thoroughly.
3. Coat the chicken wings with the seasonings each piece is covered.
4. Put an aluminum foil on the base of the Air Fryer, similar to how you cover a baking tray. Add the chicken and sprinkle the remaining seasoning over the chicken.
5. Set the timer for 15 minutes. Flip the wings over and continue cooking 15 additional minutes at 392ºF.
6. Serve piping hot.

Fried Chicken

Ingredients:

2 chicken thighs - no skin and bones

3 sprigs fresh parsley

Garlic powder – for dusting

Salt and black pepper if desired

½ a lemon

Chili flakes to our liking

1 to 2 sprigs fresh rosemary

Preparation Steps:

1. Rinse the thighs and dry with paper towels.
2. Preheat the Air Fryer: Program the temperature setting to 356°F.
3. Clean the rosemary sprigs and remove the stems. Chop or mince the parsley.
4. For the Marinade: Combine the salt, pepper, garlic powder, rosemary leaves, parsley, chili flakes, and lemon juice. Add the thighs and marinate overnight in the refrigerator.
5. Air fry for 12 minutes.

   Note: Time may vary depending on the thickness/size of the thighs.

Orange Chicken Wings

Yields: 2 Servings

Ingredients:

1 orange – zest and juice

6 chicken wings

1 ½ tbsp. Worcestershire sauce

1 tbsp. sugar

Herbs: Sage, mint thyme, basil, parsley, oregano, or other favorites

Pepper to taste

Preparation Steps:

1. Prepare the wings: Pour the juice and zest into a bowl. Add the rest of the ingredients and rub in. Let it marinate for 30 minutes.
2. Set the temperature on the Air Fryer to 356°F.
3. Add the wings to the fryer basket for 20 minutes.
4. Remove the wings from the fryer and discard excess zest.
5. Brush half of the sauce over the wings. Arrange them back in the Air Fryer and cook another 10 minutes.
6. Add the wings to a serving platter and enjoy.

Turkey

Mozzarella Turkey Rolls

Yields: 4 Servings

Ingredients:

1 sliced tomato

4 slices turkey breast

½ c. freshly chopped basil

1 c. sliced mozzarella

For Tying: 4 chive shoots

Preparation Steps:

1. Heat up the Air Fryer to 390F.
2. On each slice of turkey - add a slice of cheese, tomato, and basil.
3. Roll up each one and tie them with the chive shoot.
4. Add to the Air Fryer for 10 minutes. Serve warm.

Roast Turkey Reuben

Yields: 2 Servings

Ingredients:

4 slices rye bread

8 slices skinless – roasted turkey breast

4 tbsp. coleslaw

8 slices Swiss cheese

2 tbsp. each of each:

 -Salted butter

 -Russian dressing

Preparation Steps:

1. Prepare two slices of the bread on one side with butter and lay them butter side down on the cutting board.
2. Prepare the Sandwiches: In layers, arrange the turkey, cheese, coleslaw, and Russian dressing on top of two slices of bread. Fold them together to make one sandwich.
3. Add the sandwich to the Air Fryer basket. (You may want to make 2 batches.)
4. Push 'm' and choose the bake icon setting it to 310°F for 12 minutes.
5. After six minutes, flip the sandwich, and continue until browned.
6. When done, slice and serve.

Turkey & Avocado Burrito

Yields: 2 Servings

Ingredients:

8 slices cooked turkey breast

4 eggs

Pepper & Salt – to taste

4 tbsp. salsa

½ c. sliced avocado

¼ c. mozzarella cheese -grated

½ sliced red bell pepper

2 tortillas

Preparation Steps:

1. Program the Air Fryer temperature to 390°F.
2. Whisk the eggs with the pepper and salt.
3. Spray the Air Fryer tray with some non-stick cooking oil. Add the eggs. Cook for 5 minutes. Add the eggs to the tortillas.
4. Layer the turkey, avocado, peppers, cheese, and salsa. Roll it up slowly.
5. Spray the fryer and arrange the burritos in the basket. Cook for 5 minutes.
6. Serve warm and enjoy even when you're on the go.

Turkey Breast with Maple Mustard Glaze

Yields: 6 Servings

Ingredients:

1 (5 lb.) whole turkey breast

2 tsp. olive oil

1 tsp. of each:

-Salt

-Dried thyme

-Butter

½ tsp. of each:

-Black pepper

-Smoked paprika

-Dried sage

¼ c. maple syrup

2 tbsp. Dijon mustard

Preparation Steps:

1. Before you begin, warm up the fryer to 350°F.
2. Prepare the breast with a coat of olive oil.
3. Mix the sage, thyme, pepper, salt, and paprika as a rub. Coat the turkey with this mix.
4. Add the breast in the fryer basket and air fry for 25 minutes. Flip it over on the other side and fry another

12 minutes. It's cooked when the internal temperature reaches 165°F.

5. Meanwhile, whisk the butter, syrup, and mustard in a saucepan. Turn the breast again and brush the glaze over the breast. Give it a final 5 minutes until crispy brown.

6. Cover it with a foil tent for 5 minutes. Slice and serve.

Seafood

Cajun Shrimp

Yields: 4 to 6 Servings

Ingredients:

½ tsp. Old Bay seasoning
16-20 (1 ¼ lb.) tiger shrimp
¼ tsp. each:
 -Smoked paprika
 -Cayenne pepper
1 pinch of salt
1 tbsp. olive oil

Preparation Steps:

1. Warm up the Air Fryer to 390°F.
2. Mix all of the ingredients.
3. Coat the shrimp with the oil and spices.
4. Place the shrimp in the basket and cook for five minutes.
5. Enjoy with rice!

Cod Sticks

Yields: 5 Servings

Ingredients:

1 lb. Cod

3 tbsp. milk

2 large eggs

2 c. breadcrumbs

¼ tsp. salt

½ tsp. black pepper

1 c. almond flour

Preparation Steps:

1. Set the Air Fryer temperature to 350°F.

2. Prepare 3 bowls; one for the almond flour; one for milk and eggs; and another for pepper, salt, and breadcrumbs.

3. Dip the sticks in the flour, egg mixture, and the breadcrumbs.

4. Place in the basket for 12 minutes. Halfway through the air frying process, pause and shake the basket.

5. Serve with your favorite sauce.

Crab Herb Croquette

Yields: 6 Servings

Ingredients:

1 lb. crab meat

2 egg whites

1 c. breadcrumbs

1/4 c. chopped of each:

 -Onion

 -Red pepper

4 tbsp. of each:

 -Mayonnaise

 -Sour cream

2 tbsp. chopped celery

1 tsp. olive oil

1/2 tsp. of each:

-Parsley

-Lime juice

1/4 tsp. of each:

 -Salt

 -Chives

 -Tarragon

Preparation Steps:

1. Combine the salt and breadcrumbs in one container. In another bowl whisk the egg whites. Add the rest of the ingredients in another container.
2. Make the croquettes and dip into the spices mixture, the egg whites, and lastly the breadcrumbs.
3. Arrange in the Air Fryer basket and cook for 18 minutes.
4. Serve while hot.

Salmon Croquettes

Yields: 4 Servings

Ingredients:

1 lb. can red salmon

1 c. breadcrumbs

1/3 c. vegetable oil

½ bunch chopped parsley

2 eggs

Preparation Steps:

1. Set the Air Fryer at 392ºF.
2. Drain and mash the salmon. Combine with the beaten eggs and parsley.
3. In another dish, mix the oil and breadcrumbs.
4. Make 16 croquettes with the mixture and coat with the breadcrumbs.
5. Arrange in the preheated basket. Cook for 7 minutes.
6. Enjoy for lunch or when you want something new.

Beef

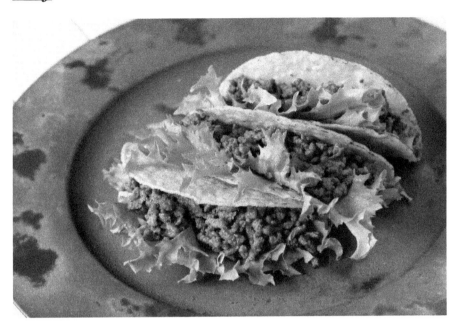

Beef & Bacon Taco Rolls

Yields: 2 Servings

Ingredients:

2 c. ground beef

4 turmeric coconut wraps/ wraps of your choice

½ c. bacon bits

1 c. of each:

  -Tomato salsa

  -Shredded Monterey Jack Cheese

To Taste - with the beef taco spices:

-Garlic powder

-Chili powder

-Black pepper

Preparation Steps

1. Warm up the fryer to 390°F.
2. Season the beef with the spices.
3. Add all the goodies into the wraps.
4. Roll them and arrange in the Air Fryer.
5. Air fry for 15 minutes and serve.

Beef Empanadas

Yields: 4 Servings

Ingredients:

½ green pepper

2 cloves of garlic

1 small onion

1 lb. ground beef

1 pkg. empanada shells

¼ c. tomato salsa

½ tsp. cumin

1 egg yolk

Pepper & Sea salt – to your liking

1 tbsp. olive oil

Preparation Steps:

1. Deseed and dice the green pepper. Peel and mince the onion and garlic.
2. Oil a sauté pan. In high heat setting, cook the ground beef until brown and drain the grease. Add the onions and garlic. Continue to fry for 4 minutes.
3. Except for the milk, egg, and shells, add in the rest of the ingredients. Cook on low heat for 10 minutes.
4. Make an egg wash with the yolk and milk.
5. Add the meat to half of the rolled dough brushing the edges with the wash. Fold it over and seal with the fork then brush with the wash.
6. Add it to the basket.
7. Repeat the process until all are done.
8. Cook in the Air Fryer for 10 minutes at 350°F.

Beef Stew

Yields: 6 Servings

Ingredients:

10 oz. beef short ribs

2 tsp. butter

½ tsp. chili flakes

1 tsp. turmeric

¼ tsp. salt

1 c. chicken stock

½ onion

1 green pepper

1 garlic clove

4 oz. of each:

  - Kale

  -Green peas

Preparation Steps:

1. Set the temperature of the Air Fryer to 360°F.
2. Melt the butter in the fryer basket and add the ribs.
3. Sprinkle with the chili flakes, salt, and turmeric. Cook for 15 minutes.
4. Prep the Veggies: Remove the seeds and chop the green pepper and kale. Dice the onion and mince garlic clove.
5. Once the ribs are done, pour in the chicken stock, the peppers and onions. Add in the peas and the minced clove of garlic.
6. Stir well and add the chopped kale. Cook 8 more minutes.
7. Let the stew steep for a short while to blend in all the delicious flavors.

8.   Serve and enjoy!

Cheeseburger Mini Sliders

Yields: 3 Large Servings

Ingredients:

6 slices cheddar cheese

1 lb. ground beef

6 dinner rolls

Black pepper and Salt

Preparation Steps:

1. Set the temperature of the Air Fryer to 390°F.

2. Form 6 patties and flavor with the pepper and salt.

3. Cook the burgers in the basket for 10 minutes.

4. Take them from the cooker and add the cheese.

5. Return them to the Air Fryer for an additional minute or until the cheese melts.

Country Fried Steak

Yields: 1 Serving

Ingredients:

1 (6 oz.) sirloin steak

3 beaten eggs

1 c. of each:

-Flour

-Panko

1 tsp. of each:

-Salt

-Pepper

-Garlic powder

-Onion powder

6 oz. ground sausage

2 tbsp. flour

2 c. milk

Preparation Steps:

1. Set the temperature in the Air Fryer to 370°F.
2. Use a meat mallet to beat the steak until thin.
3. Add the seasonings to the panko.
4. Dredge the beef with the flour, egg, and panko.
5. Arrange the steak in the basket. It should be cooked for about 12 minutes. Remove the steak.
6. For the Gravy: Cook the sausage. Drain but save 2 tablespoons of the sausage drippings in the pan. Mix in the flour along with the sausage and mix well.
7. Pour the milk and mix until thickened. Add a sprinkle of pepper and cook for approximately three more minutes.
8. Enjoy.

Inside Out Cheeseburgers

Yields: 4 Servings

Ingredients:

3/4 lb. lean ground beef

3 tbsp. minced onion

2 tsp. yellow mustard

4 tsp. ketchup

8 dill pickle chips

4 slices cheddar cheese

To Taste:

-Freshly cracked black pepper

-Salt

Preparation Steps:

1. Program the Air Fryer to 370°F.
2. Break the cheese into small bits.
3. In a large container, mix the ketchup, ground beef, pepper, salt, and mustard. Make four patties. Place the cheese and patties side by side.
4. Flatten the patty and place four pickle chips on it. Add a layer of cheese then add another patty. Press the meat together tightly to keep the contents intact while cooking.
5. Arrange the burgers in the basket and air-fry for 20 minutes. Flip after about 10 minutes.
6. Serve with a bun, tomato, and some lettuce.

Maggi Hamburgers for Lunch

Yields: 4 Servings

Ingredients:

1 lb. of lean ground beef

1 tsp. of each:

-Maggi seasoning sauce

-Dried parsley

1-2 drops liquid smoke

1 tbsp. Worcestershire sauce

½ tsp. of each:

-Ground black pepper

-Salt substitute

-Dried oregano

-Onion powder

-Garlic powder

Preparation Steps:

1. Program the temperature setting in the Air Fryer to 350°F.
2. Combine all the seasonings in a small dish then add in the beef. Mix well until perfectly combined.
3. Prepare four patties and arrange them on the tray together. Cook for 10 minutes, depending on the desired doneness. You don't need to flip them.
4. Serve and enjoy.

Roast Beef for Sandwiches

Yields: 6 Servings

Ingredients:

1 tsp. dried thyme

½ tsp. of each:

-Garlic powder

-Oregano

1 tbsp. olive oil

2 lb. round roast

Preparation Steps

1. Heat up the Air Fryer to 330°F.
2. Combine the spices. Brush the oil over the beef and rub in the spice mixture.
3. Add to a baking dish and place in the fryer for 30 minutes. Turn it over and continue cooking 25 more minutes. Let it sit for a few minutes before slicing.
4. Serve with your bread of choice or eat it as it is.

Taco Fried Egg Rolls

Yields: 8 Servings

Ingredients:

1 lb. lean (93%) ground beef

½ of an onion – chopped

16 egg roll wrappers

1 can - Cilantro Lime Ro-Tel

½ pkg. taco seasoning

½ can fat-free refried black beans

1 tbsp. olive oil

1 c. reduced-fat Mexican cheese

½ c. frozen whole kernel corn

Preparation Steps:

1. Program the fryer temperature to 400°F.
2. Warm up a frying pan using the med-high heat setting to sauté the garlic and onions. Toss in the beef, seasoning pack, salt, and pepper.
3. Add in the corn, beans, and Ro-tel.
4. Prepare the wrappers on a flat surface. Glaze the wrappers with a brush dipped in water along the edges to make the roll easier to close.
5. Load them up and use two wrappers for this amount of beef. Sprinkle each one with some cheese. Roll them up and tuck in each end. Spray with olive oil.
6. Add to the Air Fryer and cook for 8 minutes. Flip the rolls over and cook for another 4 minutes. The time may vary – depending on the size of the cooker.

Suggestion: You don't need to double wrap the rolls but

it will be a bit messy.

More Delicious Dishes

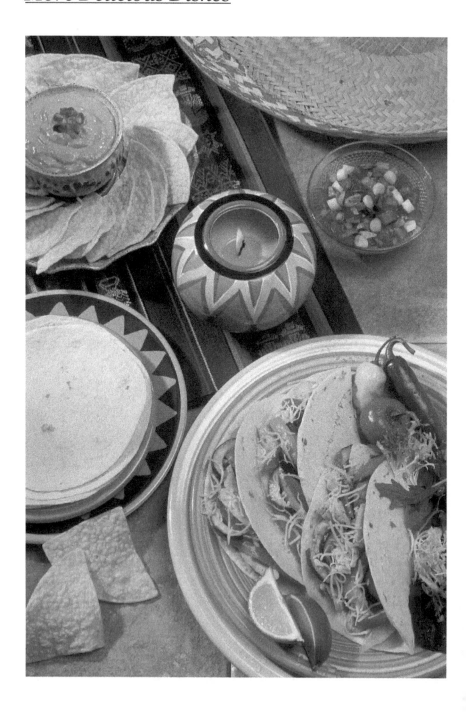

Bean Burritos

Yields: 4 Servings

Ingredients:

1 can – 15 oz. – beans

1/4 tsp. of each:

  -Garlic powder

  -Paprika

  -Chili powder

1 c. grated cheddar cheese

To Your Liking: Salt & Pepper

4 tortillas

Preparation Steps:

1. Warm up the fryer until it reaches 350°F.
2. Prepare a baking dish with a layer of parchment paper.
3. Whisk together the chili powder, garlic powder, paprika, salt, and pepper in a small dish.
4. Prepare the tortillas on a flat surface. Put the beans and top with the cheese. Sprinkle with the spices.
5. Roll the tortillas and add to the baking tray dish.
6. Place in the Air Fryer and cook 5 minutes. Serve.

Shrimp & Rice Frittata – Gluten-Free

Yields: 4 Servings

Ingredients:

4 eggs
1/2 c. of each:
  -Cooked rice
  -Baby spinach
  -Cooked shrimp
  -Grated Monterey Jack cheese
1/2 tsp. dried basil
Pinch of salt

Also Needed: 6x6x2 baking dish

Preparation Steps:

1. Warm up the Air Fryer to 320°F.
2. Lightly spray the pan with cooking spray.
3. Whisk the eggs with the basil and salt until frothy.
4. Combine the shrimp, rice, and spinach and add to the pan. Pour in the egg mixture and sprinkle with the cheese.
5. Bake for 14-18 minutes until browned.

Stromboli

Yields: 4 Servings

Ingredients:

1 pkg. (12-oz.) refrigerated pizza crust

¾ c. Mozzarella shredded cheese

3 c. shredded cheddar cheese

1 egg yolk

1 tbsp. milk

3 oz. roasted red bell peppers

1/3 lb. sliced cooked ham

Preparation Steps:

1. Warm up the Air Fryer to 360°F.
2. Roll the dough until it is ¼-inch thick.
3. Layer in the peppers, ham, and cheese on half of the dough and fold to seal.
4. Combine the milk and eggs. Brush the mixture on the dough.
5. Put the Stromboli dough in the basket and set the timer for 15 minutes. Check it every five minutes or so—flip the Stromboli to the other side for thorough cooking.

Zucchini Roll-Ups

Yields: 2 Servings

Ingredients:

1 c. goat cheese

3 zucchinis

Sea salt to taste

¼ tsp. black pepper

1 tbsp. olive oil

Preparation Steps:

1. Warm up the Air Fryer to 390°F.
2. Slice the zucchini thinly – lengthwise. Brush each strip with the oil.
3. Mix the cheese with the salt and pepper. Scoop onto the zucchini strips, roll, and fasten with a toothpick.
4. Arrange in the fryer and prepare for 5 minutes. Serve and enjoy.

Chapter 3: Dinner Time!

Seafood

Breaded Fried Shrimp

Yields: 4 Servings

Ingredients:

3 tbsp. or 1 egg white

1 lb. raw shrimp

½ c. all-purpose flour

¾ c. panko breadcrumbs

1 tsp. paprika

Pepper and salt to your liking

McCormick's Grill Mates Montreal Chicken Seasoning

Cooking spray

Ingredients for the Sauce:

2 tbsp. Sriracha

1/3 c. plain non-fat Greek yogurt

1/4 c. sweet chili sauce

Preparation Steps:

1. Peel and devein the shrimp.
2. Warm up the Air Fryer to 400°F.
3. Add the seasonings to the shrimp.
4. Use three bowls for the flour, egg whites, and breadcrumbs, egg whites.
5. Dip the shrimp into the flour, the egg, and lastly the breadcrumbs.
6. With the cooking spray, lightly spray the shrimp and add to the fryer basket for four minutes. Flip the shrimp over and cook for another four minutes. Watch the last few minutes to prevent burning.
7. For the Sauce: Combine all of the ingredients and combine thoroughly.

Cajun Salmon

Yields: 1-2 Servings

Ingredients:

1 salmon fillet – 3/4-in. thick

1/4 lemon - juiced

For Coating: Cajun seasoning

Optional: Sprinkle of sugar

Preparation Steps:

1. Warm up the Air Fryer to 356°F. The process usually takes about 5 minutes.
2. Rinse and pat the salmon dry. Thoroughly coat the fish with the Cajun seasoning mix.
3. Arrange the fillet in the fryer for 7 minutes with the skin side up.
4. Serve with a sprinkle of the lemon.

Catfish

Yields: 3 Servings

Ingredients:

4 catfish fillets

1 tbsp. olive oil

¼ c. seasoned fish fry

Preparation Steps:

1. Heat up the Air Fryer to 400°F.

2. Rinse the fish and pat them dry with a towel.
3. Empty the seasoning into a large zipper type baggie. Add the fish and shake to cover each fillet. Spray the fillets with some oil and add to the basket.
4. Cook for ten minutes, flip, and cook for ten more minutes. Flip once more and cook for 2 to 3 minutes.
5. Once desired crispiness is reached, remove, and serve.

Coconut Shrimp

Yields: 3 Servings

Ingredients:

12 - large shrimp
1 c. of each:
  -Flour
  -Breadcrumbs
  -Egg white
  -Coconut – Unsweetened (+) Dried
1 tbsp. cornstarch

Preparation Steps:

1. Warm the Air Fryer to reach 350°F.

2. Prepare a shallow platter and combine the breadcrumbs and coconut. In another bowl, mix the cornstarch and flour. Place the egg white in another small bowl.
3. Coat the shrimp with the egg white, flour, and lastly, the breadcrumbs.
4. Arrange in the fryer basket for 10 minutes.
5. Serve with your favorite sides or enjoy as a quick snack.

Cod Steaks with Ginger

Yields: 2 Servings

Ingredients:

2 slices large cod steaks

¼ tsp. turmeric powder

1 pinch of salt & pepper

½ tsp. of each:

-Ginger powder

-Garlic powder

1 tbsp. plum sauce

Ginger slices

1 part Kentucky Kernel Seasoned flour (+) 1 part cornflour

Preparation Steps:

1. Dry the cod steaks with paper towels and marinate with the ginger powder, pepper, salt, and turmeric powder for 2 to 3 minutes.
2. Lightly coat each of the steaks with the cornflour and Kentucky Flour mix.
3. Place the cod steaks into the Air Fryer. Warm up the Air Fryer to 356°F for 15 minutes. Increase to 400°F for 5 minutes. (Time may vary depending on the size of the cod.)
4. Prepare the sauce in a wok. Brown the ginger slices and remove from the heat. Add the plum sauce. If desired, dilute the sauce with a small amount of water.
5. Serve the steaks with a drizzle of the tasty sauce.

Halibut Steak with a Teriyaki Glaze Sauce

Yields: 3 Servings

Ingredients:
1 lb. Halibut steak

Ingredients for the Marinade:
2/3 c. low-sodium soy sauce
½ c. Mirin Japanese cooking wine
¼ c. of each:

-Sugar

-Orange juice

2 tbsp. lime juice

¼ tsp. each:

-Ground ginger

-Crushed red pepper flakes

1 smashed garlic clove

Preparation Steps:

1. Warm up the Air Fryer to 390°F.
2. Mix all the marinade components in a pan. Bringing to a boil. Lower the heat to medium and then cool.
3. Pour half of the marinade in a plastic bag with the halibut and zip it closed. Refrigerate for 30 minutes.
4. Remove and cook the halibut for 10 to 12 minutes. Brush some remaining glaze mixture on the steak.
5. Serve over the top a bed of rice. Add a little basil or mint for extra flavor.

Italian Cod Fillets

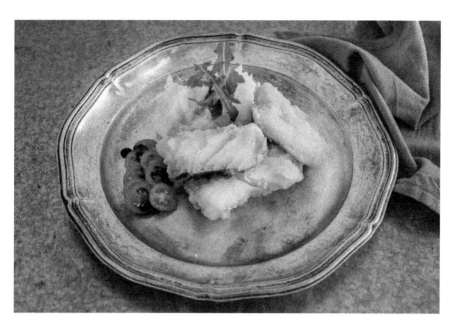

Yields: 4 Servings

Ingredients:

4 cod fillets

1 Italian pepper

4 minced cloves of garlic

1 tsp. of each:

  -Cayenne pepper

  -Dried basil

1/2 tsp. dried basil

1/4 tsp. of each:

  -Ground black pepper

  -Fine salt

1/2 c. of each:

  -Non-dairy milk – your choice

-Fresh Italian parsley

Preparation Steps:

1. Program the temperature in the Air Fryer to 380°F.
2. Spritz a baking dish with a little cooking oil.
3. Season the fillets with the cayenne, salt, and pepper.
4. Puree the rest of the fixings in a food processor.
5. Add the puree to the cod fillets.
6. Air fry for 10-12 minutes until the cod flakes easily

Oregano Clams

Yields: 4 Servings

Ingredients:

2 doz. shucked clams

4 tbsp. melted butter

1 c. unseasoned breadcrumbs

3 minced garlic cloves

1 tsp. dried oregano

¼ c. of each:

  -Chopped parsley

  -Grated parmesan cheese

1 c. sea salt

Preparation Steps:

1. Heat the Air Fryer until it reaches 400°F.
2. Mix the oregano, breadcrumbs, parmesan cheese, parsley, and melted butter in a mixing container.
3. Add a heaping tablespoon of the crumbs mixture to the clams.
4. Fill the insert of the Air Fryer with the salt, arrange the clams inside, and air fry for three minutes.
5. Garnish with some lemon wedges and fresh parsley.

Sake Glazed Salmon

Yields: 4 Servings

Ingredients:

4 fillets of flounder

1 1/2 tbsp. dark sesame oil

2 tbsp. sake

1 tbsp. grated lemon rind

1/4 c. soy sauce

2 minced garlic cloves

1 tsp. brown sugar

To Your Liking:

 -Cracked mixed peppercorns

 -Sea Salt

To Serve: Freshly chopped chives

Preparation Steps:

1. Combine all of the fixings in a mixing container (except the chives).
2. Marinate the fillets for 2 hours in the fridge.
3. Preheat the fryer to 360°F.
4. Remove the fish from the fridge and cook in the Air Fryer 10-12 minutes. Flip about halfway through the cycle.
5. Pour the marinade into a pan using the med-low heat setting. Stir until it's thickened.
6. Serve the founder with the glaze and some fresh chives.

Salmon Patties

Yields: 6-8 Servings

Ingredients:

1 salmon portion (7 oz.)

3 large russet potatoes

1/3 c. frozen veggies - parboiled and drained

2 dill sprinkles

Dash of salt and pepper

1 egg

Ingredients for the Coating:

Breadcrumbs

Olive oil spray

Preparation Steps:

1. Set the Air Fryer to 356°F.
2. Peel and chop the potatoes into small bits and boil for about ten minutes.
3. Mash and place in the fridge to chill.
4. Grill the salmon for five minutes, flake it apart and set it to the side.
5. Combine all the ingredients and shape into patties.
6. Evenly coat with the breadcrumbs and spray with olive spray.
7. Cook in the Air Fryer for ten to twelve minutes.

Pork

Bacon-Wrapped Pork Tenderloin

Yields: 4-6 Servings

Ingredients:

3-4 bacon strips

1 pork tenderloin

1-2 tbsp. Dijon mustard

Preparation Steps:

1. Coat the tenderloin with the mustard and wrap with the bacon.
2. Set the Air Fryer at 360°F for 15 minutes. Flip and cook 10-15 more minutes.
3. Serve with your favorite sides.

Balsamic & Raspberry Smoked Pork Chops

Yields: 4 Servings

Ingredients:

4 smoked bone-in pork chops

2 large eggs

1/4 c. of each:

 -2% milk

 -All-purpose flour

1 c. of each:

 -Japanese – panko breadcrumbs

 -Finely chopped pecans

1/3 c. balsamic vinegar

2 tbsp. of each:

 -Seedless raspberry jam

 -Brown sugar

1 tbsp. thawed frozen orange juice concentrate

Preparation Steps:

1. Heat up the Air Fryer to 400°F. Spritz the basket with cooking spray.
2. Whisk the milk and eggs in one dish. In another dish, combine the pecans and breadcrumbs.
3. Dip each pork chop in the flour. Shake off the excess then, dip into the egg mix.
4. Place in the fryer in single layers. Cook for 12-15 minutes. Turn about halfway through the cooking cycle.
5. Combine the rest of the fixings in a small saucepan. Bring to a boil.

6. Simmer 6-8 minutes until thickened.

7. Serve.

BBQ Pork Ribs

Yields: 2 Servings

Ingredients:

1 lb. pork ribs

3 tbsp. BBQ sauce

1 tbsp. honey

2 chopped garlic cloves

1 tsp. of each:

  -Sesame oil

  -Soy sauce

  -Black pepper

  -Salt

1/2 tsp. mixed spice

Preparation Steps:

1. Combine the sesame oil, salt, pepper, soy sauce, garlic, honey, mixed spices, and barbecue sauce.

2. Chop the ribs to fit in the fryer.

3. Add the ribs to the marinade. Marinate for 2 hours.

4. Warm the Air Fryer to 350°F. It should take about 5 minutes.

5. Arrange the ribs in the fryer basket and cook for 15 minutes.

6. Flip them over and continue cooking for another 15 minutes.

7. Serve.

Breaded Pork Chops

Yields: 6 Servings

Ingredients:

6 (3/4-inch) center-cut boneless chops

1 large egg

3/4 tsp. kosher salt

1/2 c. panko crumbs

1/3 c. crushed cornflakes

1 1/4 tsp. sweet paprika

2 tbsp. grated parmesan cheese

1/2 tsp. of each powder:

  -Onion

  -Garlic

1/4 tsp. chili powder

1/8 tsp. Ground black pepper

Preparation Steps:

1. Warm up the Air Fryer until it reaches 400°F. Lightly spray the basket with cooking oil spray.
2. Shake the salt over the chops.
3. Mix the cornflake crumbs, panko, the kosher salt, pepper, and chili powder in a container.
4. Whisk the egg in another container and dip the pork. Then coat the pork in the crumb mixture.
5. Add to the basket. Spritz both sides of the chops with oil before browning. Prepare two batches.
6. Cook 12 minutes, flipping halfway through the cycle.

Chinese Pork Ribs

Yields: 6 Servings

Ingredients:

4 minced cloves of garlic

2 lb. pork ribs

1 tbsp. of each:

-Soy Sauce

-Honey

2 tbsp. of each:

-Hoisin sauce

-Char Siu Sauce

-Sesame oil

-Minced ginger

Preparation Steps:

1. Preheat the Air Fryer to 330°F.
2. Whisk all the fixings (except for the meat.)
3. Arrange the ribs in a container and cover with the sauce. Marinate for 4 hours.
4. Place the ribs in the hot fryer with the sauce and cook for 40 minutes.
5. Increase the temperature to 350°F. Cook 10 more minutes and serve.

Crispy Mustard Pork Tenderloin

Yields: 4 Servings

Ingredients:

1 lb. pork tenderloin

2 tbsp. Dijon mustard

1 minced garlic clove

1/2 tsp. dried basil

1 c. soft breadcrumbs

2 tbsp. olive oil

To Your Liking:

  -Freshly cracked black pepper

  -Sea salt

Preparation Steps:

1. Use a meat mallet to pound the pork until they're 3/4-inch thick. Season with the pepper and salt. Slice into 1-inch slices.
2. Coat with the mustard and sprinkle with the basil and garlic.
3. Warm up the Air Fryer to 390°F.
4. Combine the oil with the breadcrumbs on a platter and coat the tenderloin.
5. Arrange in the fryer basket and cook for 12-14 minutes. The meat temperature should reach 145°F internally.
6. Serve right away.

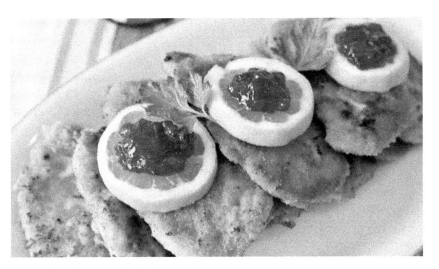

Herbed Pork & Potatoes

Yields: 2 Servings

Ingredients:

2 lb. pork loin

2 large diced potatoes

1/2 tsp. of each:

  -Freshly ground black pepper

  -Salt

  -Pepper flakes

  -Garlic powder

1 tsp. dried parsley

Preparation Steps:

1. Combine the spices (pepper flakes, garlic powder, black pepper, salt, and parsley).
2. Warm up the Air Fryer until it reaches 370°F.
3. Arrange the potatoes and pork in the fryer; next to each other. Shake in the spices. Cook for 20 to 25 minutes.
4. When done let it cool for a few minutes before slicing.
5. Serve when ready in equal portions.

Lemon Pork Tenderloin

Yields: 4 Servings

Ingredients:

1 lb. pork tenderloin
1 tbsp. of each:
  -Olive oil
  -Lemon juice
  -Honey
1/2 tsp. of each:
  -Dried marjoram
  -Grated lemon zest
Pinch of each:
  -Freshly cracked black pepper
  -Salt

Preparation Steps:

1. Slice the pork into 1/2-inch slices.
2. Combine the lemon juice, honey, olive oil, salt, pepper, marjoram, and lemon zest in a small container. Pour over the pork slices and coat well.
3. Preheat the Air Fryer to 400°F to roast.
4. Arrange the slices in the fryer basket and cook for 10 minutes. The pork should be 145°F on the meat thermometer to ensure doneness.

Tip: If you're short of time, go to the market and get a pre-marinated tenderloin.

Roast Pork Loin with Red Potatoes

Yields: 2 Servings

Ingredients:

2 lb. pork loin
2 large red potatoes
1 tsp. of each:
-Pepper
-Salt

-Parsley

½ tsp. of each:

-Red pepper flakes

-Garlic powder

Balsamic glaze from cooking

Preparation Steps:

1. Dice the potatoes. Combine all the seasonings and sprinkle over the potatoes and loin.
2. Arrange the pork and then the potatoes in the air fryer.
3. Secure the top and choose the roast button. Set the timer for 25 minutes.
4. When done, let it cool for several minutes before slicing.
5. Meanwhile, pour the roasted potatoes into the serving dishes.
6. Slice the loin into 4 to 5 sections. Use a balsamic glaze over the pork.

Southern Fried Pork Chops

Yields: 4 Servings

Ingredients:

4 pork chops

3 tbsp. buttermilk

1/4 c. all-purpose flour

To Taste:

-Pepper

-Seasoning salt

Cooking Spray

Preparation Steps:

1. Set the temperature on the Air Fryer to 380°F.
2. Rinse and pat dry the chops. Season with the pepper and salt.
3. Drizzle the chops with the buttermilk and place in a Ziploc-type bag with the flour. Toss well. Marinate for 30 minutes.
4. Arrange the chops in the fryer. (Stacking is okay.) Spritz with the cooking oil spray.
5. Air fry for 15 minutes. Flip after the first 10 minutes.
6. Enjoy while piping hot.

Chapter 4: Beef & Other Dinner Specialties

Beef

Beef & Potatoes

Yields: 4 Servings

Ingredients:

1 lb. ground beef

3 c. mashed potatoes

2 eggs

2 tbsp. garlic powder

1 c. sour cream

Black pepper – to your liking
Pinch of salt

Preparation Steps:

1. Let the Air Fryer warm until it reaches 390°F.

2. Combine all the fixings in a mixing container. Mix well and place in a heat-safe dish.
3. Place in the fryer for 2 minutes.
4. Serve and enjoy.

Beef Schnitzel

Yields: 1 Serving

Ingredients:

2 tbsp. olive oil

1 thin beef schnitzel

½ c. gluten-free breadcrumbs

1 egg

Preparation Steps:

1. Warm up the Air Fryer a couple of minutes until 356°F.
2. Combine the oil and breadcrumbs in a shallow bowl.
3. Whisk the egg in another mixing bowl.
4. Dip the beef into the egg, and then the breadcrumbs. Arrange in the basket of the Air Fryer.
5. Fry 12 minutes and serve.

Cheeseburger Patties

Yields: 6 Servings

Ingredients:

1 lb. ground beef

Black pepper

Salt

6 slices cheddar cheese

Preparation Steps:

1. Program the Air Fryer to 350°F.
2. Combine the fixings and shape into 6 burgers.
3. Air fry for 10 minutes and enjoy!

Meatloaf

Yields: 4 Servings

Ingredients:

4.5 lb. ground beef

Breadcrumbs – if homemade, use one slice of bread

1 tsp. Worcestershire sauce

3 tbsp. tomato ketchup

1 large onion – diced

1 tbsp. of each:

-Basil

-Oregano

-Parsley

Salt and pepper

Preparation Steps:

1. Program the Air Fryer temperature to 356°F.
2. Toss the beef into a large mixing container and add in the herbs, onion, Worcestershire sauce, and ketchup. Mix well for about 4 minutes and add the breadcrumbs. Combine well.
3. Add the meatloaf to the baking dish and place in the fryer. Cook for 25 minutes.

Air-fried Steak

Yields: 1 Serving

Ingredients:

1 (1 to 1 1/2-inch) beef steak

Olive oil

To Your Liking:

Pepper and salt

Preparation Steps:

1. Warm up the fryer to 350°F.
2. Cover the steak with the oil and season with the pepper and salt.
3. Arrange the prepared beef in the frying tray and cook 3 minutes on each side.
4. Serve when steak is done to your liking.

Rib Steak

Yields: 2 Servings

Ingredients:

2 lb. rib steak

1 tbsp. of each:

 -Olive oil

-Steak rub (see next recipe)

Preparation Steps:

1. Before cooking, heat up the Air Fryer to 400°F.
2. Season the steak with the oil and rub.
3. Put it in the fryer basket for 14 minutes. Flip the meat after 7 minutes.
4. Let it rest for at least 10 minutes.
5. Slice and serve.

Spicy Rub for Steak

Ingredients:

2 tbsp. granulated sugar

1 tbsp. packed brown sugar

1 ½ tbsp. each:

  -Ground cumin

  -Chili powder

  -Paprika

  -Garlic powder

1 tsp. each:

  -Onion powder

  -Salt

-Ground black pepper

-White pepper

Preparation Steps:

1. Combine all the fixings and coat your favorite meats.

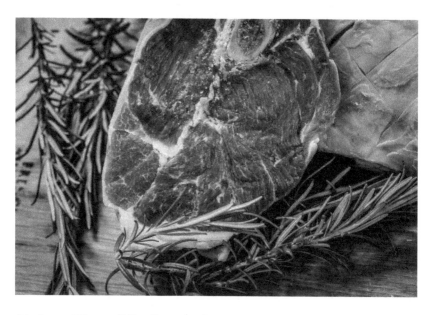

Spicy Shredded Beef

Yields: 8 Servings

Ingredients:

2 lb. beef steak

1 tsp. of each:

-Thyme

-Salt

-Ground black pepper

-Mustard

-Dried dill

4 c. chicken stock

3 tbsp. butter

1 peeled garlic clove

1 bay leaf

Preparation Steps:

1. Heat the Air Fryer ahead of time to 350°F.
2. Whisk the egg and add the stevia, baking powder, and butter.
3. Reserve 1 teaspoon of the almond flour and add the rest to the mixture. Knead until it's smooth but not sticky.
4. Layer the fryer basket with parchment paper and add the prepared crust. Flatten and place the berries on top. Sprinkle with (1 teaspoon) the almond flour.
5. Prepare the pie in the Air Fryer for 20 minutes and remove when it's golden brown.
6. Chill and slice for your awaiting guests. Add a tasty salad and enjoy.

More Dinner Delights

Lamb Meatballs

Yields: 4 Servings

Ingredients:

1 lb. ground lamb

1 egg white

4 oz. turkey

½ tsp. salt

2 minced garlic cloves

2 tbsp. parsley

1 tbsp. of each - chopped:

 -Coriander

 -Mint

1 tbsp. olive oil

Preparation Steps:

1. Heat the Air Fryer to 320°F.
2. Combine all the fixings in a mixing container. Mix well and shape into small meatballs.
3. Arrange in the Air Fryer and cook for 15 minutes.
4. When ready, enjoy with your favorite sauce or side dish.

Chapter 5: Side Dishes & Veggies

Side Dishes

Ham & Tomato Stuffed Mushrooms

Yields: 3 Servings

Ingredients:

3 Portobello mushrooms

1 tsp. minced garlic

1 med. onion

3 tbsp. grated mozzarella cheese

1 tbsp. olive oil

2 slices chopped ham

1 tomato

1 green pepper

¼ tsp. pepper

½ tsp. sea salt

Preparation Steps:

1. Warm up the Air Fryer to 320°F.

2. Dice the tomato, onion, and green pepper. Wash, dry, and remove the stems from the mushrooms. Drizzle with oil and set aside.
3. Combine the pepper, salt, cheese, tomato, onion, garlic, bell peppers, and ham.
4. Stuff into the mushroom caps.
5. Add the mushrooms to the Air Fryer for 8 minutes.

Mediterranean Veggies

Yields: 4 Servings

Ingredients:

1 green pepper

1 large of each:

 -Parsnip

 -Cucumber

¼ c. cherry tomatoes

1 med. carrot

2 tbsp. of each:

-Garlic puree

-Honey

6 tbsp. olive oil - divided

1 tsp. mixed herbs

Pepper and salt – to taste

Preparation Steps:

1. Chop the cucumber and green pepper and add to the Air Fryer.
2. Peel and dice the carrot and parsnip and add to the Air Fryer along with the whole cherry tomatoes.
3. Drizzle Fryer with 3 tablespoons of oil and cook at 356°F for 15 minutes.
4. Mix the rest of the ingredients in an Air Fryer-safe baking dish.
5. Once the veggies are done, add to the marinade and shake well. Give it a sprinkle of pepper and salt and cook at 392°F for another 5 minutes.
6. Serve and enjoy. You can also add some honey and sweet potatoes to the mixture for a tasty change of pace.

Roasted Veggie Pasta Salad

Yields: 6-8 Servings

Ingredients:

4 oz. brown mushrooms

1 red onion

1 yellow squash

1 zucchini

1 each bell peppers

 -Red

 -Green

 -Orange

Pinch of Fresh ground pepper and salt

1 tsp. Italian seasoning

1 c. grape tomatoes

½ c. pitted Kalamata olives

1 lb. cooked Rigatoni

¼ c. olive oil

2 tbsp. fresh chopped basil

3 tbsp. balsamic vinegar

Preparation Steps:

1. Preheat the Air Fryer to 380°F.
2. Prep the Veggies: Slice the squash and zucchini into half-moons. Dice the peppers into large chunks and slice the red onion. Slice the tomatoes and olives in half.
3. Put the mushrooms, peppers, red onion, squash, and zucchini in a large container. Drizzle with some of the oil. Toss well. Sprinkle in the pepper, salt, and Italian seasoning.

4. Place in the Air Fryer until the veggies are soft (ensure it doesn't get mushy), usually about for 12 to 15 minutes. For even roasting; shake the basket about halfway through the cooking cycle.

5. Combine the roasted veggies, olives, cooked Rigatoni, and tomatoes, in a large container; mix well. Add the vinegar, and toss. (Use as little oil as possible, just enough to coat the vegetables.)

6. Keep it refrigerated until ready to serve. Add the fresh basil right before serving.

Roasted Winter Veggies

Yields: 6 Servings

Ingredients:

4 celery stalks

1 parsnip

2 red onions

1 butternut squash

To Your Liking: Pepper and salt

1 tbsp. of each:

   -Olive oil

  -Fresh thyme needles

Preparation Steps:

1. Peel and chop the parsnips, celery, and remove the seeds from the squash. Dice the squash.
2. Warm up the Air Fryer to 390°F.
3. Toss all the fixings together and arrange in the fryer basket.
4. Fry for 20 minutes. Shake the basket about halfway through the cycle.

Twice Baked Loaded Air-Fried Potatoes

Yields: 2 Servings

Ingredients:

4 rashers of bacon

1 tsp. olive oil

1 potato

1 tbsp. each of each:

-Finely chopped green onion

-Unsalted butter

2 tbsp. heavy cream

¼ tsp. salt

1/8 tsp. black pepper

Preparation Steps:

1. Cook the bacon about 10 minutes. Chop into ½-inch pieces. Reserve the fat. Finely chop the onions.
2. Coat the potato with the oil and add to the Air Fryer basket. Set the temperature to 400°F for 30 minutes. Add a little more oil to the fryer, turn the potato, and cook for another 30 minutes.
3. Let it cool off for a minimum of 20 minutes.
4. When cooled, slice the potato lengthwise. Scoop out the starchy flesh, leaving about ¼-inch borders for the filling.
5. Whisk together the scooped potato flesh with the bacon fat, bacon bits, ¼ cup of the cheese, 1 ½ tsp. of the onions, pepper, salt, butter, and lastly the cream. Combine well.
6. Scoop the mixture into the prepared skins. Garnish with the cheese and place them in the Air Fryer.
7. Cook for 20 minutes or until the tops are browned, and the cheese is melted. Sprinkle the rest of the onions on top of the potato and serve.

Just Veggies

Avocado Fries

Yields: 2 Servings

Ingredients:

1 large avocado

1 beaten egg

½ c. breadcrumbs

½ tsp. salt

Preparation Steps:

1. Program the Air Fryer to 390°F.
2. Peel and remove the pit, and slice the avocado.
3. Prepare 2 shallow dishes; one with the breadcrumbs and salt; and one with the beaten egg.
4. First, dip the avocado into the egg then the breadcrumbs.
5. Add to the Air Fryer for 10 minutes.
6. Serve anytime you want a delicious side dish or an appetizer.

Baked Potatoes

Yields: 3 Servings

Ingredients:

3 Russet or Idaho baking potatoes

1 tbsp. of each:

-Salt

-Minced garlic

1 tsp. parsley

1-2 tbsp. olive oil

Preparation Steps:

1. Wash the potatoes thoroughly and poke holes in each one using a fork.
2. Oil and sprinkle the potatoes with the seasonings.
3. Add them to the Air Fryer basket and fry for 35 to 40 minutes.
4. Garnish with some sour cream and fresh parsley.

Broccoli

Yields: 2-4 Servings

Ingredients:

2 lbs. broccoli crowns

2 tbsp. olive oil

½ tsp. black pepper

1 tsp. kosher salt

2 tsp. grated lemon zest

1/3 c. Kalamata olives

¼ c. shaved parmesan cheese

6 c. water

Preparation Steps:

1. Cut away the stems of the broccoli and slice 1 to 1-1/2-inch florets. Remove the pits and cut the olives in half.
2. Using high heat, fill a medium pan with the water. Bring it to a boil. Toss in the florets and boil for 3-4 minutes. Remove and drain. Add the pepper, salt, and oil.
3. Program the Air Fryer to 400°F. After 3 minutes, arrange the broccoli into the basket, close the drawer, and click the timer for 15 minutes. Toss/flip at 7 minutes for even browning.
4. When done, place the broccoli in the bowl. Garnish with lemon zest, olives, and cheese. Enjoy.

Buffalo Cauliflower

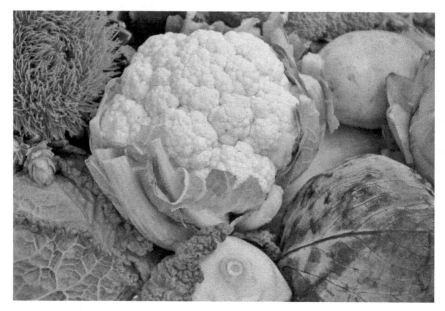

Yields: 4 Servings

Ingredients:

4 c. cauliflower florets

1 c. breadcrumbs

¼ c. each of each:

-Melted butter

-Buffalo sauce

For the Dip: Your favorite dressing

Preparation Steps:

1. Warm up the Air Fryer to 350°F.

2. Toss the butter in a microwaveable dish and cook until melted. Watch closely. Remove and whisk into the buffalo sauce.

3. Dip each of the florets into the butter mixture. Use the stem as a handle, hold it over a cup and let the excess drip away. The stem does not need to have sauce.

4. Run the floret through the breadcrumbs. Drop them into the fryer. Cook for 14 to 17 minutes.

5. Shake the basket two or three times to ensure even browning.

6. Enjoy with your favorite dip! Be sure to eat it right away because the crunchiness goes away quickly.

Cooking Tip: Reheat in the oven. Don't use the microwave or it will be mushy.

Cauliflower Rice

Yields: 3 Servings

Ingredients for Part I:

1 c. diced carrots (1½-2 carrots)

½ block extra firm or firm tofu

½ c. diced onions

2 tbsp. reduced sodium soy sauce

Ingredients for Part II:

3 c. riced cauliflower

½ c. of each:

-Finely chopped broccoli

-Frozen peas

2 minced garlic cloves

1½ tsp. toasted sesame oil – optional

1 tbsp. of each:

 -Rice vinegar

 -Minced ginger

2 tbsp. reduced sodium soy sauce

Preparation Steps:

1. Warm up the Air Fryer to 370°F.
2. Prepare the Cauliflower: Mince it into small pieces with a food processor or by hand with a box-style grater. You can also purchase the rice in the ready-made form.
3. Crumble the tofu (scrambled egg size) and add the remainder of the *Part 1* fixings. Air fry for 10 minutes. Shake once.
4. Combine the *Part II* ingredients in a large mixing container. Toss in with the fixings in the fryer. Air fry for another 2 to 5 minutes.
5. Check and shake every 2 minutes until done.

Grilled Corn

Yields: 2-4 Servings

Ingredients:

2 corn on the cob

2-3 small limes

2 tsp. paprika

Olive oil

½ c. grated feta cheese

Preparation Steps:

1. Clean the corn, by tearing away the corn silks and husks.
2. Rub the corn thoroughly with the oil and sprinkle with some paprika.
3. Warm up the fryer to 392°F.
4. Place the corn into the basket and set the timer for 12-15 minutes. Lower the time as needed if it is cooking too fast. Remove the corn from the fryer when done.
5. Grate some frozen feta cheese over the corn and drizzle with some lime juice.

Honey Roasted Carrots

Yield: 4 Servings

Ingredients:

3 c. carrots

1 tbsp. of each:

-Honey

-Olive oil

To Taste: Salt and pepper

Preparation Steps:

1. Let the Air Fryer warm up to 392°F.
2. Dice the carrots into small chunks or use baby carrots.
3. Combine the honey, oil, and carrots in a mixing dish, making sure the carrots are thoroughly coated.
4. Sprinkle pepper and salt.
5. Arrange the carrots in the Air Fryer and cook for 12 minutes.

Mushroom Melt

Yields: 10 Mushrooms

Ingredients:

10 Button mushrooms

Italian dried mixed herbs

Salt and pepper

Mozzarella cheese

Cheddar cheese

Optional Garnish: Dried dill

Preparation Steps:

1. Wash the mushrooms, remove the stems then drain.
2. Flavor with a pinch of black pepper, salt, herbs, and olive oil.
3. Heat the Air Fryer ahead of time to 356°F. (About 3 to 5 minutes should be okay.)
4. Add the mushrooms to the basket with the hollow section facing you. Sprinkle the cheese on top of each of the caps.
5. Add the mushrooms to the air fryer for 7 to 8 minutes.
6. Serve piping hot with a sprinkle of basil or other herbs.

Onion Rings

Yields: 2 Servings

Ingredients:

1 large onion

¼ c. egg whites

¼ tsp. salt

2/3 c. whole wheat panko breadcrumbs

1 tsp. of each:

-Garlic powder

-Onion powder

2 tbsp. whole wheat flour

1/8 tsp. black pepper

Preparation Steps:

1. Heat up the Air Fryer to 392°F.
2. Cut away the ends and the outer layer of the onion. Slice and separate them into rings.
3. Whisk the egg whites in a small dish.
4. Combine the seasonings and breadcrumbs in another bowl.
5. Add some flour and the rings into a plastic bag and

shake to cover the onions evenly.

6. Coat the rings with the egg whites and the breadcrumb mixture. Add the coated rings in the hot fryer.
7. Bake for 6 minutes or to your liking.

Potato Wedges

Yields: 4 Servings

Ingredients:

4 large potatoes
1 tbsp. of each:
 -Cajun spice
 -Olive oil
To Taste: Pepper and Salt

Preparation Steps:

1. Warm up the pre-oiled Air Fryer to 375°F.
2. Wash the potatoes thoroughly. Afterward, peel and chop the potatoes into wedges. Soak in water for at least 15 minutes. Soaking removes excess starch and makes for a crunchier texture when fried.

3. Remove the potatoes from the water and let dry or pat dry. Coat with Cajun spice.

4. Add to the Fryer and cook for 25 minutes. Toss midway of the cycle.

5. Enjoy with a shake of salt and pepper.

Roasted Brussels Sprouts

Yields: 4-5 Servings or approx. 1 pound

Ingredients:

1 lb. fresh Brussel sprouts

5 tsp. olive oil

1/2 tsp. kosher salt

Preparation Steps:

1. Prepare the Veggies: Trim the stems and remove any damaged outer leaves. Cut into halves, rinse, and dry. Toss with the oil and salt.

2. Set the Air Fryer temperature in advance to 390°F. Add the sprouts to the basket and cook for 15 minutes.

3. Shake the basket to make sure they cook evenly.

Roasted Corn

Yields: 4 Servings

Ingredients:

4 ears of corn
2 to 3 tsp. vegetable oil
Pepper and salt – as desired

Preparation Steps:

1. Program the temperature in the fryer to reach 400°F.
2. Remove the husks and wash the corn. Pat dry and cut to fit your Air Fryer if needed.
3. Spritz the corn with the oil and a sprinkle of salt and pepper.
4. Cook for 10 minutes and serve.

Skinny Fries

Yields: 2 Servings

Ingredients:

Salt

2-3 tsp. vegetable or olive oil

2-3 russet potatoes

Preparation Steps:

1. Slice the potatoes into ¼-inch batons using a mandolin with a julienne blade. Rinse the potatoes several times under cold water. Soak them overnight or a minimum of ten minutes.
2. Program the temperature of the fryer at 380°F.
3. Prepare two potato batches. Each batch should be enough to fill but to crowd the Fryer. Ensure that you've thoroughly drained and dried the potatoes.
4. Air fry each batch for 15 minutes, shaking once or twice. When the second batch of potatoes are almost done, toss in the first batch to reheat for a minute or so.
5. Arrange on a plate and flavor with some more salt. Serve with your choice of garnishes.

Chapter 6: Vegan Specialties

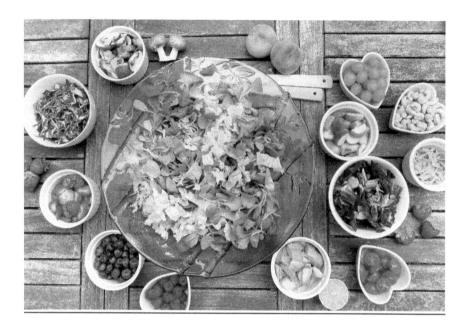

Vegan Breakfast

Apple Pancakes

Yields: 4 Servings

Ingredients:

1 3/4 c. buckwheat flour

2 tbsp. coconut sugar

1 1/4 c. almond milk

2 tsp. of each:

  -Cinnamon

-Baking powder

1/4 tsp. vanilla extract

1 apple – 1 cup

Drizzle - vegetable oil

1 tbsp. flaxseed (+) 3 tbsp. water

Preparation Steps:

1. Peel, core, and chop the apple.
2. Combine the sugar, baking powder, flour, cinnamon, and vanilla extract in a mixing bowl. Grind the flaxseed with the water and add the milk and apple.
3. Spritz oil in the fryer and spread out 1/4 of the batter. Cover and cook for 5 minutes at 360°F. Flip about halfway through the cooking cycle.
4. Continue until you have 4 excellent pancakes.

Blueberry Oats

Yields: 4 Servings

Ingredients:

2 tbsp. agave nectar

1 c. of each:

  -Steel-cut oats

  -Blueberries

  -Coconut milk

1/2 tsp. vanilla extract

Preparation Steps:

1. Lightly spray the fryer with some cooking spray. Warm the fryer until it reaches 365°F.
2. Combine all the fixings and add to the Air Fryer container.
3. Cook for 10 minutes and divide to four bowls.

Breakfast Beans Burrito

Yields: 2 Servings

Ingredients:

2 c. baked black beans

1 small avocado

1/2 red bell pepper

2 tbsp. vegan salsa

1/8 c. grated cashew cheese

To Taste: Black pepper and Salt

For Serving: Vegan tortillas

Preparation Steps:

1. Peel, pit, and slice the avocado. Slice the pepper and grate the cheese.
2. Lightly grease the Air Fryer with cooking spray.
3. Add the bell pepper, black beans, salsa, pepper, and salt.
4. Warm up the fryer to 400°F. Cook the fixings for 6 minutes.
5. Lay out the two tortillas and divide the fixings.
6. Set the temperature of the fryer at 300°F. Add the burritos to the fryer and cover. Prepare for 3 minutes more and serve.

Cheese Sandwich – Vegan Style

Yields: 1 Serving

Ingredients:

2 slices of each:

  -Vegan-friendly bread

  -Cashew cheese

2 tsp. cashew butter

Preparation Steps:

1. Warm up the Air Fryer to 370°F.
2. Spread the butter over the bread and add the cheese.
3. Slice diagonally into half.
4. Add to the fryer for 8 minutes. Flip halfway through the cycle.
5. Serve.

Chinese Breakfast Bowls

Yields: 4 Servings

Ingredients:

12 oz. cubed firm tofu

1/4 c. coconut aminos

3 tbsp. maple syrup

2 tbsp. of each:

 -Lime juice

 -Sesame oil

1 lb. fresh Romanesco broccoli

1 red bell pepper

3 carrots

8 oz. spinach

2 c. cooked red quinoa

Preparation Steps:

1. Warm up the fryer to 370°F.
2. Do the Prep: Roughly chop the Romanesco and tear apart the spinach. Cube the tofu and dice the pepper. Prepare the quinoa.
3. Combine the tofu with the lime juice, oil, maple syrup, and aminos. Add all these to the fryer for 15 minutes. Shake often.
4. Add the carrots, spinach, bell pepper, Romanesco, and quinoa.
5. Toss and portion into four dishes and enjoy.

Cinnamon Toast

Yields: 6 Servings – 2 slices per serving

Ingredients:

12 vegan slices of bread

1/2 c. coconut sugar

Pinch of black pepper

1 1/2 tsp. of each:

  -Cinnamon powder

  -Vanilla extract

A drizzle of vegetable oil

Preparation Steps:

1. Warm up the Air Fryer to 400°F.
2. Whisk the sugar, cinnamon, oil, and pepper in a mixing container.
3. Spread the mixture over the bread and arrange in the fryer for 5 minutes.
4. Serve and enjoy!

Kale Breakfast Sandwich

Yields: 1 Serving

Ingredients:

Olive oil- for the fryer

2 tbsp. pumpkin seeds

2 c. kale

1/2 tsp. jalapeno

1 small shallot

Pinch: Salt and Pepper

1 1/2 tbsp. avocado mayonnaise

1 slice of avocado

1 halved vegan bun

Preparation Steps:

1. Prep the Veggies: Tear the kale, chop the shallot, and crush the jalapeno.
2. Warm up the Air Fryer to 360°F. Spritz with oil.
3. Toss the kale, pumpkin seeds, jalapeno, shallot, pepper, and salt. Add to the cooker for 6 minutes. Shake once during the cooking process.
4. Spread the mayo on half of the bun with the avocado and kale mixture. Add the top and serve.

Polenta for Breakfast

Yields: 4 Servings

Ingredients:

1 tbsp. coconut oil

1 c. cornmeal

3 c. water

For Serving: Maple syrup

Preparation Steps:

1. Boil water using the medium heat setting. Add the cornmeal and continue cooking for 10 minutes. Pour in the oil, stir, and cook for another 10 minutes.
2. Take away from the burner and let it cool.
3. Shape into balls by the spoonful. Place on a lined baking sheet.
4. Program the fryer to 380°F. Grease the fryer basket and add the balls. Prepare for 16 minutes. Flip halfway through the cooking process.
5. Divide and serve in four plates with a serving of syrup.

Tomato Frittata

Yields: 2 Servings

Ingredients:

3 tbsp. water

2 tbsp. flax meal

2 tbsp. chopped yellow onion

1/2 c. shredded cashew cheese

1/4 c. of each:

- Diced tomatoes

-Coconut milk

Pepper & Salt – to your liking

Preparation Steps:

1. Warm up the Air Fryer to 340°F.
2. Mix the water and flax meal together.
3. Combine the milk, pepper, salt, flax meal water, onion, and cheese with the tomatoes.
4. Pour into the pan of the fryer and cook for 30 minutes.
5. When done, divide and serve in two plates.

Vegan Lunch Specialties

Chickpea Burgers

Yields: 2 Servings

Ingredients

1 can – 12 oz. – chickpeas

3 tbsp. chopped onion

4 tsp. tomato sauce

2 tsp. mustard

8 dill pickle chips

Pepper and Salt – to taste

Preparation Steps:

1. Drain and mash the chickpeas. Add in the mustard, onion, tomato sauce, salt, and pepper.
2. Portion into four segments and flatten. Add 2 pickles to the burger and cook for 20 minutes. Flip after about 10 minutes.
3. Arrange on the buns and garnish to your liking.

Eggplant Stew

Yields: 4 Servings

Ingredients:

2 large eggplants

1 red onion

24 oz. chopped – canned tomatoes

2 large bell peppers

2 tsp. ground cumin

1 tbsp. smoked paprika

1 lemon – juiced

Pepper and salt – to your liking

1 tbsp. chopped parsley

Preparation Steps:

1. Warm up the Air Fryer to 365°F.
2. Roughly chop the eggplant and peppers and combine with the rest of the fixings. (Except the parsley.)
3. Prepare for 15 minutes and remove from the fryer.
4. Sprinkle with the parsley.
5. Chill and serve cold.

Green Beans Mix

Yields: 4 Servings

Ingredients:

4 carrots – chop

1 yellow onion

1 lb. green beans

1 tbsp. thyme

4 garlic cloves

3 tbsp. tomato paste

To Taste: Black pepper & Salt

Preparation Steps:

1. Combine the carrots, onions, green beans, garlic, salt, pepper, and tomato paste in the Air Fryer pan.
2. Warm up the fryer to 365°F.
3. Prepare for 12 minutes and remove.
4. Sprinkle in the thyme and serve.

Indian Cauliflower Mix

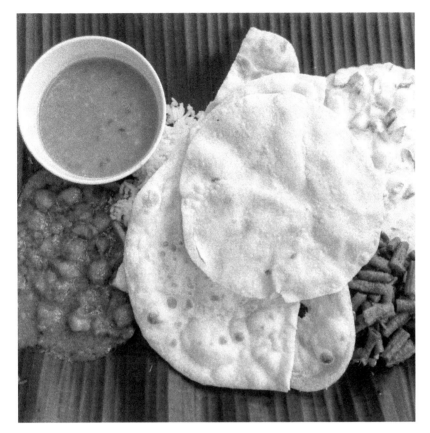

Yields: 4 Servings

Ingredients:

3 c. cauliflower florets

1/2 c. vegetable stock

A drizzle of olive oil

1 1/2 tsp. red chili powder

Pepper and Salt – to your liking

1 tbsp. ginger paste

1/4 tsp. turmeric powder

2 tbsp. water

2 tsp. lemon juice

Preparation Steps:

1. Warm up the Air Fryer to 400°F.
2. Combine all the fixings in the air fryer pan. Cook 10 minutes and lower the temperature to 360°F.
3. Prepare for 10 more minutes.
4. Divide into four portions before serving.

Potato Stew

Yields: 4 Servings

Ingredients:

6 potatoes

2 carrots

1 quart of vegetable stock

Pepper & Salt – to taste

1/2 tsp. smoked paprika

1 tbsp. parsley

1 handful thyme

Preparation Steps:

1. Heat up the Air Fryer to 375°F.
2. Chop the potatoes, carrots, thyme, and parsley.
3. Combine all the fixings in the fryer and cook for 25 minutes.
4. Serve in four bowls and enjoy.

Squash Bowls

Yields: 5 Servings

Ingredients:

2 c. broccoli florets

1 large butternut squash

1 tbsp. sesame seeds

Ingredients for the Dressing:

3 tbsp. of each:

-Olive oil

-Wine vinegar

1 1/2 tbsp. stevia

1 tbsp. of each:

  -Grated ginger

  -Coconut aminos

2 minced garlic cloves

1 tsp. sesame oil

Preparation Steps:

1. Peel and roughly cube the squash and prepare the broccoli.
2. Using a blender, mix the dressing fixings.
3. Combine the squash and broccoli with the dressing and the sesame seeds.
4. Toss and cover. Prepare for 20 minutes at 370°F.
5. Serve and enjoy.

Tasty Veggie Mix

Yields: 4 Servings

Ingredients:

2 zucchinis

2 red onions

3 tomatoes

1/4 c. of each:

-Olive oil

-Black olives

1 garlic clove

1 tbsp. of each:

-Mustard

-Lemon juice

To Taste: Salt and Pepper

1/2 c. parsley

Preparation Steps:

1. Program the temperature to 370°F.
2. Do the Prep: Chop the onions and zucchini into chunks and slice the tomatoes into wedges. Pit and slice the olives, chop the parsley, and mince the garlic.
3. Combine the fixings (omit the parsley for now) into the air fryer pan. Cook for 15 minutes.
4. Serve with a garnish of parsley and enjoy.

Vegan Treats

Almond & Vanilla Cake

Yields: 8 Servings

Ingredients:

1 c. flour

2 tsp. baking powder

1 1/2 c. of each:

 -Water

 -Stevia

1/2 c. chocolate almond milk

1/4 c. (+) 2 tbsp. cocoa powder

1 tsp. vanilla extract

2 tbsp. canola oil

Preparation Steps:

1. Spray the baking pan with cooking oil spray. Heat up the Air Fryer to 350°F.
2. Combine 2 tablespoons of the cocoa, with the flour, baking powder, oil, milk, and vanilla extract in a mixing container.
3. Spread into the prepared baking pan.

4. In another mixing dish, combine the rest of the cocoa and water. Mix well and spread over the batter in the cooker.
5. Air fry for 30 minutes and set aside to cool.
6. Slice and enjoy!

Chocolate & Coconut Bars

Yields: 12 Servings

Ingredients:

2 tbsp. of each:

-Coconut butter

-Stevia

1 c. sugar-free vegan-friendly chocolate chips

2/3 c. coconut cream

1/4 tsp. vanilla extract

Preparation Steps:

1. Program the temperature setting to 356ºF.
2. Pour the cream into a bowl and combine with the butter, stevia, and chips.

3. Set aside for five minutes and stir. Mix in the vanilla.
4. Add the mixture to a lined sheet that fits in the Air Fryer.
5. Cook for seven minutes then let it cool.
6. Slice into 12 equal portions and serve.

Coffee Pudding

Yields: 4 Servings

Ingredients:

2 oz. of each:
  -Wheat flour
  -Coconut sugar
  -Flax meal (+) 2 tbsp. water – mixed together
1 tsp. baking powder
4 oz. of each:
  -Chopped dark vegan chocolate
  -Coconut butter
Juice of 1/2 orange
1/2 tsp. instant coffee

Preparation Steps:

1. Heat up the Air Fryer to 360°F.

2. Use the medium heat setting on the stovetop to heat up the coconut butter. Add the chocolate and juice. Stir well and set aside.

3. In a mixing container, combine the sugar, coffee, and flax meal. Blend with a hand mixer and add the chocolate, salt, baking powder, and flour. Stir well.

4. Pour into the greased pan and add to the Air Fryer. Prepare for 10 minutes. Serve piping hot.

Peach Cobbler

Yields: 4 Servings

Ingredients:

1/4 c. coconut sugar

4 c. peaches

1/2 tsp. cinnamon

1 1/2 c. crushed plain vegan crackers

1/4 tsp. ground nutmeg

1/4 c. stevia

1/2 c. almond milk

1 tsp. vanilla extract

Also Needed: 1 pie plate

Preparation Steps:

1. Heat up the Air Fryer to 350°F.
2. Mix the peaches with the cinnamon and sugar.
3. In another dish, combine the nutmeg, stevia, vanilla, and almond milk.
4. Spray the pie plate with cooking spray and layer the peaches.
5. Add the cracker mix to the plate and cook for 30 minutes.
6. Serve and enjoy!

Pears & Raisins Dessert

Yields: 12 Servings

Ingredients:

6 large pears
1/2 c. raisins
1/4 c. coconut sugar
1 tsp. of each:
  -Ginger powder
  -Grated lemon zest

Preparation Steps:

1. Core and chop the pears. Grate the lemon and warm up the Air Fryer to 350°F.
2. Combine all the fixings and stir. Pour the mixture into the fryer for 25 minutes.
3. Add to the desired containers and chill.
4. Enjoy when cold.

Raspberry Bars

Yields: 12 Servings

Ingredients:

1/2 cup of all:
  -Melted coconut butter
  -Swerve
  -Dried raspberries
  -Coconut oil
  -Shredded coconut

Also Needed: Food Processor

Preparation Steps:

1. Blend the dried berries together in the food processor.
2. Use a bowl that fits in the fryer.   Combine the oil, butter, coconut, Swerve, and berries. Toss them and cook for 6 minutes.
3. Once done, lay the mixture out over a lined baking sheet and store in the refrigerator for at least an hour.
4. Slice into 12 servings and enjoy whenever you have the urge for a special treat.

Simple & Sweet Bananas

Yields: 4 Servings

Ingredients:

3 tbsp. of each:
  -Coconut butter
  -Cinnamon
8 bananas
2 tbsp. flax meal (+) 2 tbsp. water – mix together
1/2 c. corn flour
1 c. vegan breadcrumbs

Preparation Steps:

1. Warm up the Air Fryer to 280°F.
2. Remove the peel of the bananas and slice into halves.
3. Warm up the butter (med-high heat) in a skillet and add the breadcrumbs. Cook for 4 minutes then add to a mixing bowl.
4. Roll the banana halves in the flour, flax meal, and breadcrumbs.
5. Arrange the prepared bananas in the fryer basket. Dust with the cinnamon sugar and cook for 10 minutes.
6. Enjoy!

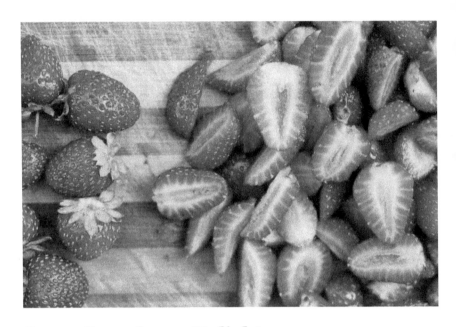

Sweet Strawberry Delight

Yields: 10 Servings

Ingredients:

2 lb. strawberries

2 tbsp. lemon juice

4 c. coconut sugar

1 tsp. of each:

  -Cinnamon

  -Vanilla extract

Preparation Steps:

1. Heat up the Air Fryer until it reaches 350°F.
2. Prepare a pan that will fit into the Air Fryer.
3. Combine the berries, coconut sugar, cinnamon, vanilla, and lemon juice. Stir gently and add to the fryer pan.
4. Cook for 20 minutes and break down into portions.
5. Serve when cold.

Vanilla & Blueberry Squares

Yields: 8 Servings

Ingredients:

5 oz. melted coconut oil

4 tbsp. stevia

1/2 tsp. baking powder

3 tbsp. flax meal (+) 3 tbsp. water – mix together

4 oz. coconut cream

1 tsp. vanilla

1/2 c. blueberries

Preparation Steps:

1. Combine the oil, flax meal, coconut cream, baking powder, stevia, and vanilla in a mixing container. Mix well with an immersion blender.
2. Fold in the berries and place to a baking dish.
3. Prepare for 20 minutes.
4. Slice when cool. Serve cold.

Chapter 7: Vegetarian Choices

Breakfast Choices

Asparagus Strata

Yields: 4 Servings

Ingredients:

4 eggs

6 asparagus spears

2 slices whole wheat bread

3 tbsp. whole milk

1/2 c. grated Swiss cheese

Pinch of salt

2 tbsp. chopped flat-leaf parsley

To Taste: Freshly cracked black pepper

Preparation Steps:

1. Warm up the Air Fryer to 330°F.
2. Cut the asparagus into 2-inch pieces and slice the bread into 1/2-inch pieces.

3. Arrange the spears of asparagus with 1 tbsp. of water in a baking pan. Place in the fryer and bake for 3-5 minutes. Take it out of the pan and drain.
4. Spray the pan with a layer of cooking oil spray.
5. Arrange the asparagus and bread chunks in the pan and set to the side.
6. Whisk the milk and eggs and mix with the salt, pepper, cheese, and parsley. Pour into the pan and bake 11-14 minutes. Cook until they're the way you like them.

Banana & Peanut Butter Sandwiches

Yields: 2 Servings

Ingredients:

2 tbsp. peanut butter
4 slices whole wheat bread
2 sliced bananas
1/4 tsp. cinnamon powder

Preparation Steps:

1. Toast the bread in the fryer for 3 to 5 minutes until browned on one side.

2. Prepare the sandwiches by putting peanut butter on one side of each bread.
3. Add the sliced bananas on the buttered side of the slices. Dust with the cinnamon and top with the remaining bread.
4. Toast for 3 minutes or so for the second side of the bread and enjoy.

Breakfast Burritos

Yields: 2 Servings

Ingredients:

1 tbsp. of each:

 -Water

 -Liquid smoke

2 tbsp. of each:

 -Tamari

 -Cashew butter

4 pieces hydrated rice paper

2 servings – vegan egg scramble

1/3 c. of each:

 -Roasted sweet potato cubes

 -Sautéed broccoli

6 stalks fresh asparagus

Handful of kale

8 strips roasted red pepper

Ingredients for the Stuffing:

1/2 tsp. oil

1 crushed clove of garlic

1 tbsp. soy sauce

2 c. cooled – cooked rice

1 diced carrot

1 c. frozen peas

1 diced onion

Preparation Steps:

1. Warm up the fryer to 350°F.
2. Whisk the cashew butter, tamari, liquid smoke, and water.
3. Combine the rest of the fixings in the rice papers. Fold, roll and dip in the tamari mixture.
4. Prepare in the air fryer for 8 to 10 minutes.

Cheesy Toast

Yields: 1 Serving

Ingredients:

1/4 c. grated cheese

2 slices of bread

1 pat butter

Preparation Steps:

1. Warm up the fryer to 392°F.
2. Spread the butter over the toast and add the cheese.
3. Add to the Air Fryer for 4-5 minutes.

Cranberry Beignets

Yields: 16 Beignets

Ingredients:

1 1/2 c. flour

1/4 tsp. salt

2 tsp. baking powder

3 tbsp. brown sugar

1/2 c. buttermilk

1/3 c. chopped dried cranberries

1 egg

3 tbsp. unsalted butter – melted

Preparation Steps:

1. Warm up the Air Fryer until it reaches 330°F.
2. Whisk the brown sugar, flour, salt, and baking soda. Mix well.
3. Stir in the cranberries.
4. In another dish combine the egg with the buttermilk.
5. Stir the mixture into the dry ingredients, until moistened.
6. Make an 8x8 square and slice into 16 sections. Cover with melted butter.
7. Prepare in batches. Layer the pieces so they don't touch in the Air Fryer.
8. Cook for 5-8 minutes. If desired, dust with some powdered sugar.

Dutch Pancake

Yields: 4 Servings

Ingredients:

3 eggs

2 – scant tbsp. unsalted butter

1/2 c. of each:

 -Milk

 -All-purpose flour

1/2 tsp. vanilla

1 1/2 c. freshly sliced strawberries

2 tbsp. confectioner's sugar

Preparation Steps:

1. Program the Air Fryer to 330°F. Prepare the pan in the basket by adding the butter.
2. In a mixing container, whisk the eggs, milk, vanilla, and flour until frothy.
3. When the butter has melted, add to the batter and bake for 12-16 minutes.
4. The pancake will collapse when removed from the Air Fryer. Top with the berries and sugar. Enjoy immediately.

5- Cheese Bread

Yields: 2 Servings

Ingredients:

1 loaf of bread

3 1/2 oz. butter

2 tsp. of each:

  -Chives

  -Garlic puree

1 oz. of each cheese – grated:

  -Edam cheese

  -Goat's

  -Mozzarella

  -Cheddar

1 oz. soft cheese

Pepper and salt – to your liking

Preparation Steps:

1. Melt the butter in a skillet. Add in the chives and garlic with the salt and pepper. Sauté for 2 minutes. Let cool slightly.
2. In a bowl, mix skillet contents and soft cheese.
3. Slice off the top of the loaf of bread and make shallow scores. Push or embed in the butter and soft cheese mixture. Sprinkle in the rest of the grated cheeses.

4. Air fry for 4 minutes and serve with your favorite dish or on its own.

Glazed Doughnuts

Yields: 2 Servings

Ingredients:

2 c. powdered sugar

1 can biscuit dough

1/4 c. milk

Preparation Steps:

1. Warm up the Air Fryer to 390°F.
2. Combine the milk and sugar. Stir to dissolve.
3. Cut out the center of the biscuits using a cookie cutter.
4. Spritz the pan with some cooking spray and add the mixture. Fry for 5 minutes.
5. Remove and coat with the hot sugar glaze.

Lemony Blueberry Muffins

Yields: 12 Servings

Ingredients:

2 1/2 c. self-rising flour

1/2 c. of each:

 -White sugar

 -Full-cream milk

1/4 c. vegetable oil

2 Eggs

1 1/2 c. blueberries

2 lemons – juiced & zested

1/4 tsp. of each:

   -Lemon extract

  -Vanilla extract

Also Needed: Muffin tin

Preparation Steps:

1. Program the Air Fryer to 360°F.
2. Combine all the dry fixings (except the berries or zest). In another mixing container, mix the wet ones.
3. Combine both mixtures and fold in the berries and lemon zest. Scoop into the muffin tins.
4. Bake for 12 minutes. Cool on a rack before serving.

Monkey Bread

Yields: 4 Servings

Ingredients:

1 can refrigerated biscuits – 8 oz.

1/4 c. white sugar

1/8 tsp. nutmeg

1/2 tsp. cinnamon

3 tbsp. of each:

  -Brown sugar

  -Melted unsalted butter

Also Needed: 6-by-6-by-2-inch pan

Preparation Steps:

1. Program the Air Fryer to 350°F.
2. Prepare each of the biscuits by slicing them into quarters.
3. Mix the nutmeg, cinnamon, brown and white sugar.
4. Dip each of the quarters in the melted butter and into the sugar mixture.
5. Arrange in the pan and air fry/bake for 6-9 minutes.

6. Cool for 5 minutes before serving. Use caution because the sugar is *hot*.

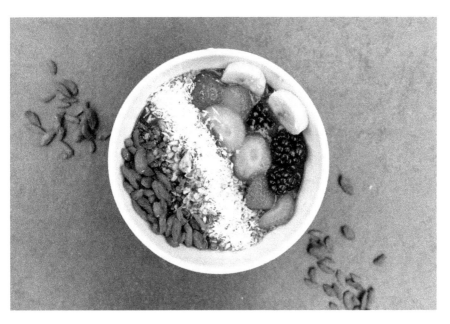

Pecan & Cranberry Granola

Yields: 4 Servings

Ingredients:

2 c. rolled oats

1/2 tbsp. canola oil

3/4 c. unsalted chopped pecans

1/4 tsp. ground cinnamon

1/8 tsp. salt

1/2 tsp. vanilla extract

1/8 c. of each:

  -Pure maple syrup

  -Dried cherries

Preparation Steps:

1. Combine all the fixings except for the cherries. Cook in the air fryer for 7 minutes.
2. Mix in the dried cherries then cook for another minute.
3. Enjoy with a hot beverage for an early morning 'pick-me-up.'

Strawberry Tarts

Yields: 9 Servings

Ingredients:

8 oz. plain flour

3 1/2 oz. butter

3/4 oz. castor sugar

Water as needed

18 tsp. strawberry jam

Preparation Steps:

1. Warm up the Air Fryer to 360°F.
2. Mix the sugar, flour, and butter in a dish until it looks like breadcrumbs. Add enough water to make a firm pastry dough. Knead.
3. Spritz 9 pastry cases and add the pastry on the sides and bottom. Spoon in 2 teaspoons of the jam.
4. Prepare in the Air Fryer for 10 minutes.

Lunch and Dinner Specialties

Cauliflower Steak

Yields: 3 Servings

Ingredients:

1 purple cauliflower head
1/2 of each – thinly sliced:
  -Yellow onion
  -Bell pepper
1 tbsp. olive oil
To Your Liking:
  -Old Bay Seasoning

-Salt

Preparation Steps:

1. Spritz the cauliflower with oil and season with the Old Bay and salt.
2. Warm up the Air Fryer to 375°F.
3. Add to a baking dish and sprinkle the pepper. Layer the onion and spritz with a bit of oil.
4. Bake for 25 minutes.

Cheese Burst Macaroni Sandwich

Yields: 1 Serving

Ingredients:

4 tbsp. macaroni and cheese

1 whisked egg

2 slices white bread

3/4 oz. cheddar cheese

Salt & Pepper – as needed

Preparation Steps:

1. Program the Air Fryer to 360F.
2. Add the cheddar cheese with the macaroni and cheese in layers on the bread. Add a slice of bread on the top and cut diagonally.
3. Use the beaten egg to brush the outer portion of the bread slices and give it a shake of pepper and salt to your liking.
4. Prepare for 5 minutes per side and enjoy.

Cheesy Tomato Sandwich

Yields: 1 Serving

Ingredients:

1 slice of cheese

2 slices of bread

4 tomato slices

1 tsp. butter

Pepper – to your liking

Preparation Steps:

1. Put the sandwich together and add the butter to the top.
2. Cook for 5 minutes. Flip it then butter the topside during the last minute of the cooking cycle.

Chili Butternut Squash

Yields: 4 Servings

Ingredients:

1 squash – in chunks – no seeds

2 tsp. cumin seeds

1 tbsp. olive oil

A pinch of chili flakes

1 bunch freshly chopped coriander

3/5 c. of plain Greek yogurt – approx.

1 1/2 oz. toasted pine nuts

Preparation Steps:

1. Prepare the squash and toss with the seasonings (cumin seeds and chili flakes) and oil.
2. Warm up the Air Fryer to 375°F.

3. Cook the mixture for 20 minutes. Toss about 10 minutes into the cooking cycle.
4. Serve with the yogurt, coriander, and nuts.

Crispy Spanish Potatoes

Yields: 3 Servings

Ingredients:

1 tbsp. water
1 1/2 lb. small red potatoes
1 tsp. of each:
  -Tomato paste
  -Smoked Spanish paprika
  -Hot smoked paprika
1/2 tbsp. brown rice flour
1/2 tsp. of each:
  -Salt
  -Garlic powder

Preparation Steps:

1. Quarter and boil the potatoes until tender.
2. Combine the water and tomato paste. Mix with the rest of the fixings except for the potatoes.

3. Now, add the potatoes to the tomato mixture and combine with the rest of the fixings.
4. Warm up the Air Fryer for at least 3 minutes.
5. Prepare the potatoes for 12 to 20 minutes. Shake about halfway through the cycle.

Potato Tacos

Yields: 4 Servings

Ingredients:

1 c. leftover mashed potatoes
1/2 c. shredded cheddar cheese
4 warmed corn tortillas
For the Garnish: Salsa of your choice

Preparation Steps:

1. Warm up the Air Fryer to 392°F.
2. Prepare each tortilla with equal portions of the potato mash. Sprinkle with the cheese.
3. Arrange in the fryer for 18 to 20 minutes.
4. Serve with the salsa and a smile.

Roasted Rhubarb & Carrots

Yields: 4 Servings

Ingredients:

2 tsp. walnut oil

1 lb. of each:

  -Rhubarb

  -Heritage carrots

1/2 c. walnut halves

1/2 tsp. stevia

1 orange – zest & sections

Preparation Steps:

1. Mix the chopped carrots with the oil and add to the fryer to cook for 20 minutes (375°F).
2. Add the nuts, chopped rhubarb, and stevia. Cook 5 more minutes.
3. Combine the orange sections and the orange zest and serve over the meal.

Soya Manchurian

Yields: 5-6 Servings

Ingredients:

1 thinly sliced bell pepper
1 c. of each:
  -Soya chunks
  -Spring onions
1 tsp. ginger garlic paste
2 tsp. of each:
  -Gram flour
  -Corn flour
1 tbsp. of each:
  -Soy sauce
  -Tomato ketchup
  -Chili sauce
3 tsp. olive oil - divided
To Taste:
  -Black pepper
  -Salt

Preparation Steps:

1. Warm up the Air Fryer to 180°F.
2. Chop the onions and slice the bell pepper. Soak and boil the soya chunks.
3. Combine the chunks with 2 teaspoons of the oil with the gram flour. Mix well and cook in the Air Fryer for 8 minutes.
4. In a pan, warm the rest of the oil with the bell pepper, onions, and ginger paste for 2 minutes. Combine the corn flour with enough water to make it runny and add to the pan. Simmer for 15 minutes.
5. Add the sauces, pepper, and salt. Simmer for another 5 minutes to thicken.
6. Serve with a topping of spring onions.

Spicy Stuffed Okra

Yields: 4 Servings

Ingredients:

8.75 oz. okra – sliced lengthwise
2 tsp. of each:
  -Cumin
  -Chili powder
  -Coriander powder

-Lime juice

Salt to taste

Pinch of turmeric

1 tsp. of each:

  -Oil

  -Chaat masala or Masala

1/2 c. chickpea flour

Preparation Steps:

1. Heat up the Air Fryer to 360°F.
2. Mix all the fixings (except the okra) and mix well to form a paste.
3. Stuff the sliced okra and prepare in the fryer for 7 minutes.
4. Serve and enjoy anytime.

Stuffed Bell Pepper

Yields: 6 Servings

Ingredients:

1 diced of each:

  -Carrot

  -Potato

-Onion

-Vegan bread roll

6 bell peppers

1/2 c. peas

2 tsp. herb mixture

1/3 c. grated vegan cheese

Preparation Steps:

1. Remove the tops and discard the pith and seeds of the peppers. Dice the veggies.
2. Combine everything but the pepper and grated cheese in a mixing container. Stuff the peppers.
3. Prepare in the Air Fryer for 5 minutes. Sprinkle with cheese and fry another 5 minutes until browned.

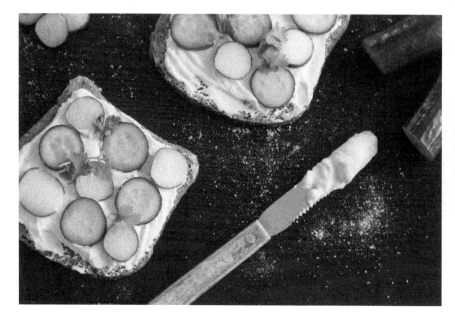

Veggies on Toast

Yields: 4 Servings

Ingredients:

1 c. cremini or button sliced mushrooms

1 red bell pepper

1 small sliced yellow squash

2 green onions

4-6 slices Italian or French bread

Olive oil – For misting

1/2 c. soft goat cheese

2 tbsp. softened butter

Preparation Steps:

1. Warm up the Air Fryer until it reaches 330°F.
2. Mix the onions, squash, mushrooms, and red peppers in the Air Fryer. Spritz with some cooking oil.
3. Roast for 7-9 minutes. Shake once during the process.
4. Remove the veggies and set to the side.
5. Add butter to one side of the bread. Arrange in the fryer, butter-side up.
6. Toast for 2-4 minutes. Spread the goat cheese on the bread, add the veggies, and serve.

Yogurt Veggie Salad

Yields: 4 Servings

Ingredients:

3 diced eggplants

2 zucchinis

2 sweet peppers

2 garlic cloves

1 tbsp. of each:

-Balsamic vinegar

-Olive oil

8 3/4 oz. low-fat yogurt

1 – 8 oz. - glass tomato juice

1 diced tomato

1 tsp. of each:

  -Sugar

  -Salt

Preparation Steps:

1. Mix the olive oil, tomatoes, and cloves of garlic together.
2. Cook in the Air Fryer for 15 minutes.
3. Add the zucchinis and eggplant and fry for another 10 minutes.
4. Season with the pepper and continue cooking for an additional 10 minutes.
5. Add the 'fried' mixture in with the rest of the fixings and serve.

Zucchini – Yellow Squash & Carrots

Yields: 2-4 Servings

Ingredients:

1/2 lb. carrots

1 lb. of each:

 -Zucchini

 -Yellow squash

6 tsp. olive oil - divided

1/2 tsp. ground white pepper

1 tsp. kosher salt

1 tbsp. roughly chopped tarragon leaves

Preparation Steps:

1. Warm up the fryer to 400°F.
2. Prep the Veggies: Cut away the ends of the squash and zucchini and slice into 3/4-inch moons. Peel and slice the carrots into 1-inch cubes.
3. Combine and toss the carrots with 2 teaspoons of the oil. Arrange the carrots in the basket and cook for 5 minutes.
4. Meanwhile, drizzle the rest of the oil, salt, and pepper with the squash and zucchini in another container.
5. Once the carrots are done (buzzer goes off); add the other fixings and set the timer for 30 minutes more. Toss several times to promote even browning.

6. Remove from the Air Fryer when the time has elapsed. Toss with the tarragon and serve warm.

Snacks & Desserts

Chocolate Brownies

Yields: 4 Servings

Ingredients:

4 1/2 oz. of each:
  -Butter
  -Castor sugar
2/3 c. milk
2 eggs
1 3/4 oz. chocolate
2 tsp. vanilla essence
3 1/2 oz. self-rising flour
3/4 c. brown sugar

Preparation Steps:

1. Warm up the Air Fryer to 360°F. Prepare a dish with a spritz of oil that will fit into the frying unit.

2. In a saucepan, melt the butter and chocolate. Blend in the brown sugar, eggs, flour, and vanilla. Place on the oiled dish and cook for 15 minutes.

3. Use the medium heat setting on the stove to combine the sugar and water. Increase the temperature and stir for 3 minutes until it's a light brown. Let it cool for 2 minutes. Blend in the milk and butter.

4. Cool slightly, and cut the brownies into four squares and top it off with the delicious sauce.

Ice Cream Sandwiches

Yields: 2 Servings

Ingredients:

3/4 oz. butter
4 wholemeal bread slices
2 tbsp. diced almonds
2 ice cream scoops

Preparation Steps:

1. Spread a scoop of the ice cream over the bread slice and toss some almonds on it.
2. Place the top on the sandwich and cut out with a cookie cutter. Pinch the sides together. Repeat the process and freeze.
3. Warm up the fryer to 360°F.
4. Butter both sides of the frozen ice cream.
5. Cook for 3 minutes each side in the Air Fryer.

Indian Corn Vadas

Yields: 2 Servings

Ingredients:

2 tbsp. corn

2 green chilies

1/2 c. split brown chickpeas

1/2 tsp. ginger garlic paste

1 crumbled fresh slice of bread

To Your Liking: Salt

Pinch of baking soda

1 tsp. oil.

Preparation Steps:

1. Warm up the Air Fryer for about 5 minutes until it reaches 360°F.
2. Combine the chickpeas, corn, and green chilies to make a paste.
3. Blend in the rest of the fixings and shape into cutlets.
4. Air fry for 8 minutes and enjoy.

Khichdi Balls

Yields: 4 Servings

Ingredients:

1 tomato

2 onions

1 bell pepper

1/2 c. of each:

  -Split brown chickpeas

  -Rice

2 green chilies

1/4 oz. cumin

1/2 tbsp. red chili powder

To Taste: Salt

Preparation Steps:

1. Program the Air Fryer to 360°F.
2. Prepare the khichdi with the rice and chickpeas. Let it cool. Combine the rest of the fixings.
3. Combine into small balls and cook for 10-12 minutes.

Sweet Potato Popcorn

Yields: 4 Servings

Ingredients:

4 tbsp. coconut milk

5 oz. sweet potatoes

1 spring onion

1 white onion

1 tsp. of each:

-Chives

-Ginger puree

-Garlic puree

Pepper and Salt – to taste

Preparation Steps:

1. Warm up the Air Fryer until it reaches 360°F.
2. Steam the potatoes 20 minutes, cool, and mash.
3. Combine the rest of the fixings. Shape into small balls and place in the Air Fryer for 20 minutes.
4. Serve with a serving of barbecue sauce.

Chapter 8: Appetizers & Snacks

Appetizers

Avocado Bacon Fries

Yields: 2 Servings

Ingredients:

1 egg

1 c. almond flour

4 bacon strips

2 large avocados

For the Fryer: Olive oil

Preparation Steps:

1. Cook the bacon and break into small bits.
2. Program the temperature of the Air Fryer to 355°F.
3. Whisk the eggs in one bowl. Add the flour with the bacon in another.
4. Slice the avocado lengthwise and dip into the eggs then the flour mixture.

5. Drizzle oil in the fryer tray and cook 10 minutes on each side or until they're the way you like them.

Bacon-Wrapped Chicken

Yields: 3 Servings

Ingredients:

1 chicken breast
1 tbsp. soft garlic cheese
6 strips unsmoked bacon

Preparation Steps:

1. Slice the chicken into 6 portions.
2. Spread the garlic cheese over each strip of bacon. Add a piece of chicken to each one. Roll and secure with a toothpick.
3. Prepare the Air Fryer for 2 to 3 minutes. Add the wraps and cook 15 minutes.
4. Serve hot.

Bacon-Wrapped Shrimp

Yields: 4 Servings

Ingredients:

1 lb. of each:

-Bacon slices

-Peeled shrimp

Preparation Steps:

1. Program the temperature of the Air Fryer to 390°F.
2. Wrap a bacon slice around each shrimp. Add to the fryer basket
3. Prepare for 5 minutes in the fryer and enjoy.

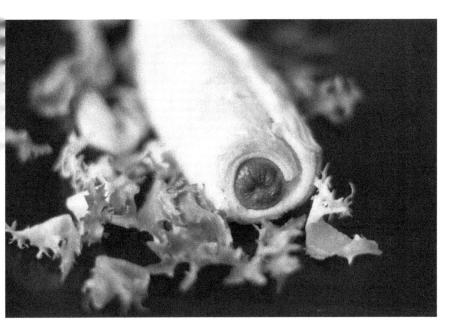

Pigs 'N' A Blanket

Yields: 4 Servings

Ingredients:

1 can (8 oz.) crescent rolls

1 pkg. cocktail hotdogs (12 oz.)

Preparation Steps:

1. Program the temperature of the Air Fryer to 330°F.
2. Drain the hot dogs and thoroughly dry them using two

paper towels.

3. Slice the dough into strips of about 1 ½ in x 1 in (rectangular).

4. Roll the dough around the franks leaving the ends open. Put them in the freezer to firm up for about 5 minutes.

5. Take them out and arrange them in the Air Fryer from 6 to 8 minutes. Adjust the temperature to 390°F. When it's hot, continue to cook for approximately 3 minutes.

Snacks

Apple Chips

Yields: 6-8 Servings

Ingredients:

6 large red apples
1 tbsp. olive oil
A pinch of cinnamon

Preparation Steps:

1. Heat up the Air Fryer to 356°F.

2. Slice the apples lengthwise and add them to the Air Fryer with the oil.
3. Cook until they are crispy or around 10 minutes.
4. Add the cinnamon, give them a toss, and enjoy.

Cheese Balls

Yields: 5 Servings

Ingredients:

1 egg
8 oz. pkg. mozzarella balls
½ c. of each:
  -Coconut flakes
  -Almond flour
To Taste:
  -Thyme
-Pepper
  -Paprika

Preparation Steps:

1. Program the heat setting on the Air Fryer to 400°F.

2. Beat the egg in one bowl while combining the spices with flour in a separate bowl.

3. Sprinkle the balls with the coconut flakes and the flour. Freeze for 5 minutes. Add to the fryer for 3 minutes and enjoy!

Chickpeas with Ranch Seasoning

Yields: 4 Servings

Ingredients:

2 tbsp. olive oil – divided

1 can – 15 oz. chickpeas

1 tsp. sea salt

1 batch homemade ranch seasoning

2 tbsp. lemon juice

Preparation Steps:

1. Warm up the fryer to 400°F.

2. Drain but don't rinse the chickpeas and add them to a bowl with 1 tablespoon of the oil and fry for 15 minutes.

3. Add the chickpeas back into the bowl and toss in the rest of the oil, salt, seasoning, and lemon juice.

4. Return mixture to the Air Fryer with the temperature

reset at 350°F for another 5 minutes

5. Serve and enjoy. The chickpeas will keep on counter for a couple of days.

Fried Pickles

Yields: 14 Pickles

Ingredients:

¼ c. all-purpose flour

1/8 tsp. baking powder

14 thinly sliced dill pickles – refrigerated & crunchy

Pinch of salt

3 tbsp. dark beer (German beer - if vegan)

2-3 tbsp. water

6 tbsp. panko breadcrumbs

2 tbsp. cornstarch

Pinch of cayenne pepper

½ tsp. paprika

For Frying: Organic canola or oil spray

¼-1/2 cup ranch dressing

Preparation Steps:

1. Use paper towels to dry the pickles. Set to the side for

later.

2. Mix the beer, two tablespoons of water, a pinch of salt, baking powder, and flour. Its consistency should be similar to waffle batter.

3. Prepare two platters. One will have the cornstarch, and the other will have a pinch of salt, the cayenne, paprika, and breadcrumbs.

4. Bread the pickles. Prepare the working surface with the pickles, cornstarch, beer batter, and panko mixture.

5. Dip each of the pickles into the cornstarch and remove excess starch. Dip each one into the batter until evenly covered. Let the excess batter drip away. Lastly, add the pickle into the panko mixture to cover all surfaces.

6. Add the finished pickles to the air fryer basket. Heat the fryer to 360°F.

7. Do this in batches, spraying each layer with some cooking oil. Check the pickles after eight minutes. If not ready, add them back and cook checking every minute.

8. Serve with the ranch dressing and enjoy!

Mozzarella Sticks

Yields: 4 Servings

Ingredients:

2 eggs

1 lb. /1 block mozzarella cheese

1 c. plain breadcrumbs

¼ c. white flour

3 tbsp. nonfat milk

Preparation Steps:

1. Set the temperature in the Air Fryer to 400°F.
2. Slice the cheese into 1/2-in x 3-in sticks.
3. Whisk the milk and egg together in one bowl. Also, provide individual dishes for the oil and breadcrumbs. Dredge the sliced cheese through the oil, egg, and breadcrumbs.
4. Place the sticks on bread tin and put them in the freezer compartment for about 1 to 2 hours.
5. Arrange them in small portions into the fryer basket (don't overcrowd). Cook for 12 minutes.

Spicy Nuts

Yields: 3 Cups

Ingredients:

1 beaten egg white

¼ tsp. ground cloves

½ tsp. ground cinnamon

Pinch of cayenne pepper

Salt to your liking

1 c. of each:

  -Pecan halves

  -Cashews

  -Almonds

Preparation Steps:

1. Mix the spices with the egg white. Warm up the Air Fryer to 300°F.
2. Toss the nuts into the mixture and shake.
3. Prepare in the Air Fryer for 25 minutes. Stir 2 to 3 times.

Chapter 9: Desserts

Blackberry Pie

Yields: 8 Servings

Ingredients:

1 large egg

2 tbsp. unsalted butter

1 tbsp. baking powder

1 scoop stevia

1 c. almond flour

½ c. blackberries

Also Needed: Parchment paper

Preparation Steps:

1. Program the temperature to the Air Fryer at 350°F.
2. Whisk the egg and add the butter, stevia, and baking powder.
3. Reserve 1 tsp. of the flour and add the rest to the mixture. Knead until smooth and not sticky.
4. Cover the fryer basket with the paper and add the dough. Flatten into the shape of a pie crust and add the

berries. Sprinkle with the rest of the almond flour on top.

5. Air fry 20 min. Chill before slicing to serve.

Blackberry Scones

Yields: 10 Servings

Ingredients:

1 c. blackberries

1/2 c. coconut flour

2 tbsp. of each combined:

  -Water

  -Flax meal

1/2 c. of each:

  -Coconut butter

  -Coconut cream

  - Almond Flour

  -5 tbsp. stevia

2 tsp. of each:

  -Baking powder

  -Vanilla extract

Preparation Steps:

1. Warm up the Air Fryer to 350°F.
2. Whisk the baking powder with the almond flour, coconut flour, and blackberries. Gently stir well.
3. Combine the flax meal mixture, cream, vanilla extract, butter, and stevia in another bowl. Mix well.
4. Combine it all and stir into a dough. Shape into ten triangles. Arrange on a baking sheet to fit in the Air Fryer.
5. Cook for 10 minutes. Serve chilled.

Cherry Pie

Yields: 8 Servings

Ingredients:

2 refrigerated pie crusts
1 can cherry pie filling - 21 oz.
1 egg yolk
1 tbsp. milk

Preparation Steps:

1. Warm up the fryer to 310°F.
2. Poke several holes into the crust after placing it into a pie plate. Let the excess to hang over the edges. Place in the Air Fryer for 5 minutes
3. Take the basket out and set the crust on the counter. Fill it with the cherries. Remove the excess crust.
4. Cut the remaining crust into 3/4-inch strips placing them as a lattice across the pie.
5. Make an egg wash with the milk and egg. Brush top of the pie.
6. Bake for 15 minutes. Serve with the ice cream of your choice.

Green Avocado Pudding

Yields: 3 Servings

Ingredients:

1 pitted avocado

5 tbsp. almond milk

3 tsp. stevia

¼ t of each:

  -Vanilla extract

  -Salt

1 tbsp. cocoa powder

Preparation Steps:

1. Preheat the Air Fryer a couple of minutes until it reaches 360°F.
2. Peel and mash the avocado. Mix with the milk, salt, vanilla extract, and stevia. Stir in the cocoa powder.
3. Prepare in the Air Fryer for 3 minutes. Chill well and serve.

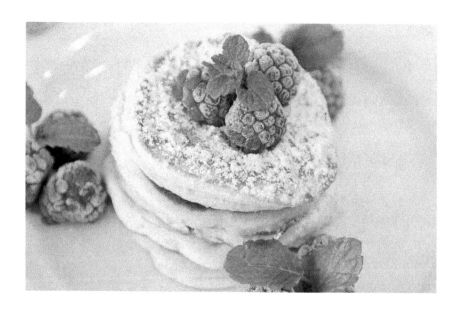

Conclusion

I hope you enjoyed every section of this book and I hope it was informative and able to provide you with all of the tools you need to achieve your goals whatever they may be.

Air Frying is one of the healthiest ways to cook and I'm positive the recipes included here will make your life easier and your meal times tastier!

If you found this book useful in any way,   please do leave a review on Amazon. I will really appreciate it!

CPSIA information can be obtained
at www.ICGtesting.com
Printed in the USA
BVHW051142230522
637799BV00011B/145